KIDNEY DISEASE DIET COOKBOOK FOR MEN

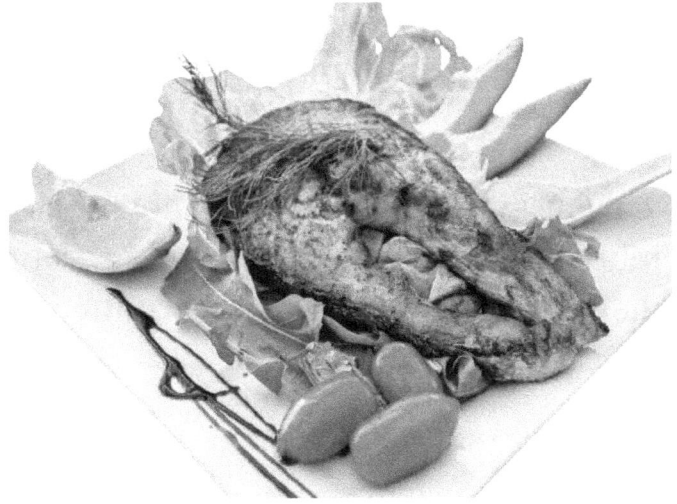

Your Complete Guide to Delicious and Nutritious Recipes to Manage Chronic Kidney Diseases

Tina Feldman

Copyright © Tina Feldman 2024

All rights reserved. No part of this publication may be reproduced, distributed, or transmitted in any form or by any means, including photocopying, recording or other electronic or mechanical methods, without the prior written permission of the publisher, except in the case of brief quotations embodied in critical reviews and certain other non-commercial uses permitted by copyright law.

Table of Contents

INTRODUCTION 7
PART 1: Understanding Kidney Disease and Its Impact on Men .. 9
   The role of kidney 9
   Types of Kidney Diseases 11
   Symptoms and Risk Factors Specific to Men 13
   Emotional and Psychological Toll of Kidney Diseases 16
   Embracing Hope and Empowerment in the Face of Kidney Challenges 19
PART 2: Meal Planning for Kidney Disease 23
   Essential Nutrients for Optimal Kidney Health 23
   Principles of Crafting a Kidney-Friendly Diet 26
   Practical Meal Planning Tips for Men Managing Kidney Disease 29
PART 3: Staying Active and Fit with Kidney Disease 33
   Debunking Exercise Myths for Men with Kidney Disease 33
   Physical Benefits of Exercise for Kidney Health 36
   Low-Impact Exercises Tailored for Kidney Health 39
   Gentle Strength Training Strategies for Men Managing Kidney Disease 42
   The Mental Health Benefits of Exercise in Kidney Disease Management 46
PART 4: HEALTHY AND DELICIOUS RECIPES 49
BREAKFAST 49
   Vegetable Omelette 49
   Greek Yogurt Parfait 50

Spinach and Mushroom Frittata 50

Banana-Oat Pancakes 51

Avocado Toast with Poached Egg 52

Quinoa Breakfast Bowl 53

Egg and Vegetable Breakfast Burrito 54

Blueberry-Almond Smoothie 55

Cottage Cheese Pancakes 55

Apple-Cinnamon Overnight Oats 56

LUNCH 57

Grilled Chicken Salad with Lemon-Tahini Dressing 57

Quinoa and Black Bean Stuffed Bell Peppers 58

Salmon and Asparagus Foil Packets 59

Turkey and Vegetable Stir-Fry 60

Vegetarian Lentil Soup 61

Mediterranean Chickpea Salad 62

Tuna Salad Lettuce Wraps 63

Eggplant and Tomato Pasta 64

Vegetable and Lentil Curry 65

Turkey and Avocado Wrap 66

DINNER 67

Grilled Lemon Herb Chicken 67

Baked Salmon with Roasted Vegetables 68

Turkey and Vegetable Stir-Fry 69

Vegetarian Chickpea and Spinach Curry 70

Lemon Garlic Shrimp Pasta 71

    Turkey Meatball and Vegetable Skewers 72

    Eggplant Parmesan 74

    Vegetable and Tofu Stir-Fry 75

    Lemon Herb Baked Cod 76

    Mushroom and Spinach Quinoa Risotto 77

DESSERT 78

    Fruit Salad with Honey-Lime Dressing 78

    Baked Apples with Cinnamon and Walnuts 79

    Mixed Berry Parfait 80

    Banana-Oat Cookies 81

    Chia Seed Pudding 82

    Peach and Yogurt Popsicles 83

    Frozen Yogurt Bark 83

    Coconut Chia Seed Pudding 84

    Chocolate Banana Smoothie 85

    Baked Pears with Cinnamon and Almonds 86

SNACKS 87

    Greek Yogurt and Berry Parfait 87

    Cucumber and Hummus Slices 88

    Apple Slices with Almond Butter 88

    Carrot Sticks with Cottage Cheese Dip 89

    Whole Grain Crackers with Tuna Salad 90

    Edamame 90

    Yogurt-Covered Pretzels 91

    Banana-Oat Energy Bites 91

- Roasted Chickpeas 92
- Vegetable Sushi Rolls 93

SMOOTHIES 94
- Berry Blast Smoothie 94
- Green Power Smoothie 95
- Banana Almond Smoothie 96
- Tropical Paradise Smoothie 97
- Peanut Butter Banana Smoothie 98
- Cherry Vanilla Smoothie 99
- Peach Raspberry Smoothie 100
- Chocolate Banana Protein Smoothie 101
- Minty Pineapple Smoothie 102
- Coconut Banana Smoothie 103

BONUS 104
- Shopping list 104

CONCLUSION 109

INTRODUCTION

Welcome to "Cooking for Kidney Health: A Diet Cookbook for Men"! This cookbook is crafted specifically to empower men who are navigating the challenges of kidney disease and seeking to take control of their health through mindful and nourishing eating habits.

For men facing kidney disease, dietary adjustments can often feel overwhelming and restrictive. However, with the right knowledge, guidance, and a dash of creativity, managing kidney health through food can be both manageable and enjoyable. That's where this cookbook comes in.

Within these pages, you'll find a collection of delicious and kidney-friendly recipes tailored to meet the unique nutritional needs of men with kidney disease. From hearty breakfast options to satisfying dinners and everything in between, each recipe is thoughtfully designed to be not only nutritious but also flavorful and satisfying.

But this cookbook is more than just a compilation of recipes. It's a comprehensive guide to understanding kidney disease and its impact on men's health. You'll find valuable information on the importance of kidney health, the different types of kidney diseases, common symptoms and risk factors specific to men, as well as the emotional and psychological toll that kidney diseases can bring. Moreover, we'll explore practical strategies for embracing hope and empowerment in the face of kidney challenges.

In addition to understanding kidney disease, we'll delve into the fundamentals of crafting a kidney-friendly diet. You'll discover essential nutrients for optimal kidney health, principles for building balanced and nourishing meals, and practical meal planning tips to make healthy eating a seamless part of your lifestyle.

Furthermore, this cookbook will debunk common myths surrounding exercise for men with kidney disease while highlighting the physical and mental health benefits of staying active. You'll find tailored exercise strategies and low-impact workouts specifically designed to support kidney health and overall well-being.

Whether you're just beginning your journey with kidney disease or you're seeking new culinary inspiration to enhance your current dietary regimen, "Cooking for Kidney Health: A Diet Cookbook for Men" is your trusted companion on the path to better health and vitality.

PART 1: Understanding Kidney Disease and Its Impact on Men

The role of kidney

The kidneys play a crucial role in maintaining overall health by performing several vital functions within the body. Here are some of the key roles of the kidneys:

- Filtration of Blood: One of the primary functions of the kidneys is to filter waste products and excess substances from the blood. Every day, the kidneys filter around 120 to 150 quarts of blood to produce about 1 to 2 quarts of urine, which contains waste products such as urea, creatinine, and excess electrolytes.

- Regulation of Fluid Balance: The kidneys help regulate the balance of fluids in the body by adjusting the amount of water excreted in urine. They ensure that the body maintains a stable internal environment, preventing dehydration or excess fluid accumulation (edema).

- Electrolyte Balance: Along with regulating fluid balance, the kidneys also play a crucial role in maintaining the balance of electrolytes such as sodium, potassium, calcium, and phosphorus in the body. Proper electrolyte balance is essential for nerve function, muscle contraction, and overall cellular function.

- Blood Pressure Regulation: The kidneys produce hormones such as renin, which helps regulate blood pressure by controlling the volume of blood and the constriction or dilation of blood vessels. They also play a role in the long-term regulation of blood pressure by influencing the balance of salt and water in the body.

- Acid-Base Balance: The kidneys help maintain the body's acid-base balance by excreting hydrogen ions and reabsorbing bicarbonate ions, which help buffer acids in the blood. This function is crucial for maintaining the body's pH within a narrow range to support optimal cellular function.

- Production of Hormones: In addition to renin, the kidneys produce other hormones such as erythropoietin (EPO), which stimulates the production of red blood cells in the bone marrow, and calcitriol (active vitamin D), which helps regulate calcium and phosphorus levels in the body.

- Detoxification: The kidneys play a vital role in detoxifying the body by filtering out toxins, drugs, and metabolic waste products from the blood and excreting them in urine. This detoxification process helps maintain overall health and prevents the accumulation of harmful substances in the body.

Types of Kidney Diseases

Kidney diseases encompass a broad spectrum of conditions that affect the structure and function of the kidneys. These diseases can range from mild and easily manageable to severe and life-threatening. Understanding the types of kidney diseases is essential for proper diagnosis, treatment, and management. Here are some of the most common types of kidney diseases:

Chronic Kidney Disease (CKD):

1. CKD is a long-term condition characterized by the gradual loss of kidney function over time. It is often associated with conditions such as diabetes, hypertension (high blood pressure), and glomerulonephritis.
2. CKD progresses through stages, with early stages often showing few or no symptoms. As the disease advances, symptoms such as fatigue, swelling (edema), and changes in urine output may become apparent.
3. Management of CKD involves lifestyle changes, medication, and sometimes dialysis or kidney transplantation in advanced stages.

Acute Kidney Injury (AKI):

1. AKI, also known as acute renal failure, is a sudden and severe decrease in kidney function that occurs over a short period. It is often caused by conditions such as severe infection, dehydration, or exposure to toxins.

2. Symptoms of AKI may include decreased urine output, swelling, nausea, and confusion. In severe cases, AKI can lead to complications such as electrolyte imbalances and fluid overload.
3. Treatment of AKI focuses on identifying and addressing the underlying cause, restoring kidney function, and preventing complications.

Glomerulonephritis:

1. Glomerulonephritis is a group of kidney diseases that affect the glomeruli, the tiny blood vessels in the kidneys responsible for filtering waste and excess fluids from the blood.
2. Types of glomerulonephritis include IgA nephropathy, membranous nephropathy, and lupus nephritis, among others.
3. Symptoms of glomerulonephritis may include blood in the urine (hematuria), proteinuria (excess protein in the urine), swelling, and high blood pressure.
4. Treatment depends on the specific type of glomerulonephritis and may include medication, immunosuppressive therapy, and lifestyle changes.

Polycystic Kidney Disease (PKD):

1. PKD is a genetic disorder characterized by the growth of cysts (fluid-filled sacs) in the kidneys, which can interfere with kidney function over time.
2. Autosomal dominant PKD (ADPKD) is the most common form and typically presents in adulthood. Autosomal recessive PKD (ARPKD) is less

common and often presents in infancy or childhood.
3. Symptoms of PKD may include abdominal pain, high blood pressure, urinary tract infections, and kidney stones.
4. Management of PKD focuses on controlling symptoms, preventing complications, and preserving kidney function through medication, lifestyle modifications, and, in some cases, dialysis or transplantation.

Kidney Stones:

1. Kidney stones are hard deposits of minerals and salts that form in the kidneys and can cause severe pain when they pass through the urinary tract.
2. Types of kidney stones include calcium stones, uric acid stones, and struvite stones, among others.
3. Risk factors for kidney stones include dehydration, certain medical conditions (such as hyperparathyroidism and gout), and dietary factors.
4. Treatment of kidney stones may involve pain management, hydration, medication to help pass the stones, and, in some cases, surgical intervention.

Symptoms and Risk Factors Specific to Men

Symptoms and risk factors for kidney disease can vary between men and women due to biological and lifestyle differences. While some symptoms and risk factors may overlap, men may experience certain symptoms or be at higher risk for specific factors. Understanding these distinctions is crucial for early detection, prevention, and management of kidney disease in men.

Symptoms Specific to Men:

Urinary Changes: Men may experience changes in urinary habits or symptoms related to urinary function. These can include:

- Changes in urinary frequency, urgency, or flow.
- Difficulty initiating urination or emptying the bladder completely.
- Pain or discomfort during urination.
- Blood in the urine (hematuria) or changes in urine color.
- Sexual Dysfunction: Kidney disease can affect hormonal balance and blood flow, potentially leading to sexual dysfunction in men. Symptoms may include erectile dysfunction, reduced libido, or other sexual health issues.

- Lower Back or Flank Pain: Pain in the lower back or sides (flanks) may indicate kidney problems, such as kidney stones or kidney infections. Men may perceive this pain differently or attribute it to other causes, such as muscle strain or injury.

- Swelling: Edema, or swelling, particularly in the legs, ankles, or feet, can be a sign of kidney dysfunction. Men may notice swelling but might not always recognize it as a symptom of kidney disease.

Risk Factors Specific to Men:

- Age: Men, particularly older men, are at increased risk for developing kidney disease. Aging can lead to changes in kidney structure and function, making older men more susceptible to kidney problems.

- Hypertension (High Blood Pressure): Men tend to have higher rates of hypertension compared to women, especially at younger ages. High blood pressure is a significant risk factor for kidney disease as it can damage the blood vessels in the kidneys over time.

- Diabetes: Men have a higher prevalence of type 2 diabetes, which is a leading cause of kidney disease. Poorly controlled diabetes can damage the kidneys' filtering units (glomeruli) and increase the risk of kidney complications.

- Smoking and Alcohol Use: Men are more likely to smoke and consume alcohol excessively, both of which are risk factors for kidney disease. Smoking and heavy alcohol consumption can impair kidney function and contribute to the development or progression of kidney problems.

- Obesity and Unhealthy Diet: Men may be more prone to obesity and unhealthy dietary habits, such as high consumption of processed foods, red meat, and sodium. These factors increase the risk of conditions like diabetes, hypertension, and metabolic syndrome, all of which can harm kidney health.

- Occupational Exposures: Certain occupations, such as those involving exposure to heavy metals, solvents, or chemicals, may pose a higher risk of kidney damage for men. Occupational hazards can contribute to the development of kidney disease over time.

- Family History: Men with a family history of kidney disease or related conditions, such as hypertension or diabetes, may have a higher genetic predisposition to kidney problems.

It's important for men to be aware of these symptoms and risk factors and to seek medical attention if they experience any concerning symptoms or have risk factors for kidney disease. Early detection and management can help prevent complications and preserve kidney function in men.

Emotional and Psychological Toll of Kidney Diseases

The emotional and psychological toll of kidney disease on men can be profound and multifaceted. Coping with the diagnosis, treatment, and lifestyle changes associated with kidney disease can significantly impact a man's mental well-being, leading to various emotional challenges. Here are some of the key aspects of the emotional and psychological toll of kidney disease in men:

- Shock and Denial: Upon receiving a diagnosis of kidney disease, men may experience feelings of shock, disbelief, or denial. The sudden realization of having a chronic condition that requires lifelong management can be overwhelming and difficult to accept. Men may struggle to come to terms with the reality of their diagnosis, leading to feelings of confusion and uncertainty about the future.

- Anxiety and Fear: Living with kidney disease can evoke feelings of anxiety and fear about the progression of the illness, potential complications, and uncertainty about the future. Men may worry about the effectiveness of treatment, the need for dialysis or transplantation, financial implications, and how the disease will impact their quality of life and independence.

- Depression and Mood Changes: Chronic illness can take a toll on mental health, leading to symptoms of depression, sadness, irritability, or mood swings. Men with kidney disease may experience feelings of hopelessness, helplessness, or loss of interest in activities they once enjoyed. Depression can affect motivation, energy levels, and the ability to cope with the demands of managing kidney disease.

- Stress and Coping Challenges: Managing the physical demands of kidney disease, such as dietary restrictions, medication management, dialysis treatments, and medical appointments, can be stressful and overwhelming. Men may struggle to cope with the daily challenges of living with a chronic illness, leading to increased stress levels and difficulty adapting to lifestyle changes.

- Body Image and Self-Esteem: Kidney disease and its treatments, such as dialysis or transplantation, can have physical effects that impact body image and self-esteem. Men may experience changes in weight, appearance, or physical functioning, leading to feelings of self-consciousness, insecurity, or dissatisfaction with their bodies. Coping with these changes and adjusting to a new sense of self can be emotionally challenging.

- Social Isolation and Relationship Strain: Kidney disease can disrupt social activities, work commitments, and relationships, leading to feelings of isolation and loneliness. Men may withdraw from social interactions or feel misunderstood by others who do not fully comprehend the impact of their illness. Relationships with family members, friends, or romantic partners may also be strained by the demands of kidney disease and its effects on daily life.

- Loss and Grief: Living with kidney disease involves adjusting to loss and grieving the loss of health, independence, and future plans. Men may mourn the loss of their former selves and struggle to accept the limitations imposed by their illness. Coming to terms with these losses and finding meaning and purpose in life despite the challenges of kidney disease can be a significant emotional journey.

It's essential for men living with kidney disease to prioritize their mental health and seek support when needed. Building a strong support network of family, friends, healthcare professionals, and peer support groups can provide emotional validation, practical assistance, and encouragement during difficult times. Engaging in self-care activities, such as exercise, relaxation techniques, hobbies, and creative outlets, can also help men manage stress, improve mood, and enhance overall well-being. Seeking professional counseling or therapy may be beneficial for addressing specific emotional challenges and developing coping strategies to navigate the emotional complexities of living with kidney disease.

Embracing Hope and Empowerment in the Face of Kidney Challenges

Embracing hope and empowerment in the face of kidney challenges is essential for individuals living with kidney disease to maintain resilience, motivation, and a positive outlook on life. While kidney disease can present significant physical, emotional, and practical challenges, adopting a mindset of hope and empowerment can help individuals navigate the journey with greater strength and resilience. Here's how individuals can embrace hope and empowerment in the face of kidney challenges:

- Education and Knowledge: Empowerment begins with understanding. Individuals with kidney disease can empower themselves by educating themselves about their condition, treatment options, and self-care strategies. By learning about kidney health, dialysis, transplantation, dietary management, and lifestyle modifications, individuals can make informed decisions, actively participate in their care, and advocate for their needs.

- Positive Mindset and Attitude: Maintaining a positive mindset and attitude is crucial for fostering hope and resilience in the face of kidney challenges. Despite the difficulties and uncertainties associated with kidney disease, focusing on the present moment, practicing gratitude, and cultivating optimism can help individuals maintain a sense of hope and perspective. Affirmations, mindfulness practices, and gratitude journaling can be helpful tools for fostering a positive mindset.

- Setting Realistic Goals: Setting realistic goals and milestones can provide a sense of purpose, direction, and accomplishment for individuals living with kidney disease. Whether it's achieving specific health goals, pursuing personal interests, or engaging in meaningful activities, setting achievable goals can foster a sense of empowerment and motivation. Breaking larger goals into smaller, manageable steps can make them feel more attainable and less overwhelming.

- Self-Advocacy and Communication: Empowerment involves advocating for one's needs, preferences, and rights. Individuals with kidney disease can empower themselves by actively participating in their healthcare decisions, asking questions, expressing concerns, and communicating openly with their healthcare team. Building a collaborative relationship with healthcare providers can ensure that individuals receive personalized care that aligns with their values and goals.

- Building a Support Network: Surrounding oneself with a supportive network of family, friends, peers, and healthcare professionals can provide invaluable encouragement, empathy, and practical assistance during challenging times. Connecting with others who understand the journey of kidney disease through support groups, online communities, or peer mentoring programs can offer emotional validation, shared experiences, and practical tips for coping and resilience.

- Embracing Lifestyle Changes: Empowerment involves taking ownership of one's health and well-being through proactive lifestyle choices. Individuals with kidney disease can empower themselves by embracing healthy habits such as following a kidney-friendly diet, engaging in regular physical activity, managing stress, getting adequate sleep, and avoiding harmful substances such as tobacco and excessive alcohol.

- Celebrating Progress and Resilience: Recognizing and celebrating personal achievements, milestones, and moments of resilience can reinforce feelings of empowerment and self-worth. Whether it's reaching a health goal, overcoming a setback, or simply persevering in the face of adversity, acknowledging one's strengths and resilience can bolster confidence and motivation.

- Seeking Professional Support: Seeking professional support from mental health professionals, counselors, or therapists can be beneficial for individuals struggling with emotional challenges, such as anxiety, depression, or grief, related to kidney disease. Therapy can provide a safe space for processing emotions, developing coping strategies, and building resilience.

PART 2: Meal Planning for Kidney Disease

Essential Nutrients for Optimal Kidney Health

Optimal kidney health relies on a well-balanced diet that includes essential nutrients while also managing intake of substances that may burden the kidneys. Here are the essential nutrients for kidney health and their roles in supporting kidney function:

1. Protein: Protein is necessary for maintaining muscle mass, supporting immune function, and repairing tissues. However, individuals with kidney disease may need to moderate their protein intake, as excessive protein consumption can strain the kidneys. High-quality sources of protein, such as lean meats, poultry, fish, eggs, dairy products, and plant-based proteins like beans and tofu, are recommended. Depending on the stage of kidney disease and individual health status, protein intake may need to be adjusted under the guidance of a healthcare professional.

2. Fluids: Adequate hydration is essential for kidney health, as it helps maintain proper kidney function, supports urinary tract health, and prevents dehydration. However, individuals with kidney disease may need to monitor their fluid intake, as excessive fluid consumption can exacerbate fluid retention and high blood pressure. Healthcare providers may recommend fluid restrictions for

individuals with advanced kidney disease or those undergoing dialysis.

3. Electrolytes: Electrolytes such as sodium, potassium, calcium, and phosphorus play vital roles in maintaining fluid balance, nerve function, muscle contraction, and bone health. Individuals with kidney disease may need to monitor their electrolyte intake, as imbalances can occur due to impaired kidney function. For example, limiting sodium intake can help manage blood pressure and fluid retention, while controlling potassium and phosphorus intake can prevent electrolyte imbalances and mineral buildup in the blood.

4. Fiber: Dietary fiber is important for promoting digestive health, regulating bowel movements, and supporting heart health. High-fiber foods such as fruits, vegetables, whole grains, legumes, and nuts can help individuals with kidney disease manage blood sugar levels, cholesterol levels, and weight. However, some high-fiber foods may also contain higher levels of potassium and phosphorus, so portion control may be necessary for individuals with kidney disease.

5. Antioxidants: Antioxidants such as vitamins C and E, beta-carotene, and selenium help protect cells from damage caused by free radicals and oxidative stress. Consuming a diet rich in fruits, vegetables, nuts, seeds, and whole grains can provide a variety of antioxidants that support overall health and kidney function. Some studies suggest that antioxidants may help reduce inflammation and

slow the progression of kidney disease, although more research is needed in this area.

6. Omega-3 Fatty Acids: Omega-3 fatty acids found in fatty fish (such as salmon, mackerel, and sardines), flaxseeds, chia seeds, and walnuts have anti-inflammatory properties that may benefit individuals with kidney disease. Omega-3 fatty acids can help reduce inflammation, lower triglyceride levels, and protect against heart disease, which is a common complication of kidney disease.

7. Vitamins and Minerals: Adequate intake of vitamins and minerals such as vitamin D, vitamin B complex, iron, and zinc is important for overall health and immune function. However, individuals with kidney disease may be at risk of vitamin and mineral deficiencies due to impaired kidney function, dietary restrictions, or medication interactions. Healthcare providers may recommend vitamin and mineral supplements to address specific deficiencies and ensure optimal nutrition.

8. Phosphorus Binders: Individuals with advanced kidney disease may need to take phosphorus binders with meals to reduce absorption of phosphorus from food and prevent hyperphosphatemia (high levels of phosphorus in the blood). Phosphorus binders should be taken as directed by a healthcare provider and may be necessary when dietary restrictions alone are insufficient to control phosphorus levels.

It's important for individuals with kidney disease to work with a registered dietitian or healthcare provider to develop a personalized nutrition plan tailored to their specific needs, stage of kidney disease, and individual health goals. A well-balanced diet that includes essential nutrients while managing intake of substances that may burden the kidneys can help support optimal kidney health and overall well-being.

Principles of Crafting a Kidney-Friendly Diet

Crafting a kidney-friendly diet involves principles aimed at supporting optimal kidney function, managing symptoms, and preventing complications associated with kidney disease. Here are the key principles to consider when designing a kidney-friendly diet:

1. Limit Sodium Intake: Reducing sodium (salt) intake is crucial for managing blood pressure and fluid retention, which are common complications of kidney disease. High sodium intake can exacerbate hypertension and fluid overload. The recommended daily intake of sodium for individuals with kidney disease is typically limited to 1,500 to 2,300 milligrams per day. To reduce sodium intake, it's essential to avoid processed and packaged foods, which are often high in sodium, and instead opt for fresh, whole foods prepared with minimal salt. Using herbs, spices, and lemon juice to flavor foods can enhance flavor without adding extra sodium.

2. Control Potassium Levels: Potassium is an electrolyte that plays a role in nerve and muscle function. However, individuals with kidney disease may need to monitor their potassium intake, as impaired kidney function can lead to hyperkalemia (high potassium levels). Foods high in potassium, such as bananas, oranges, tomatoes, potatoes, and leafy greens, should be consumed in moderation or restricted, depending on individual potassium levels and kidney function. Cooking methods such as leaching or soaking vegetables can help reduce their potassium content.

3. Manage Phosphorus Intake: Phosphorus is a mineral that can accumulate in the blood when kidney function is impaired, leading to hyperphosphatemia. High phosphorus levels can contribute to bone disease, cardiovascular complications, and other adverse health outcomes. Individuals with kidney disease may need to limit their intake of phosphorus-rich foods, such as dairy products, nuts, seeds, whole grains, and processed foods containing phosphate additives. Phosphorus binders may also be prescribed to help control phosphorus absorption from food.

4. Moderate Protein Consumption: While protein is essential for muscle repair and overall health, excessive protein intake can strain the kidneys and exacerbate kidney disease progression. Depending on the stage of kidney disease and individual health status, healthcare providers may recommend moderating protein intake to reduce the workload on the kidneys. High-quality sources

of protein, such as lean meats, poultry, fish, eggs, dairy products, and plant-based proteins like beans and tofu, are preferred. Portion control and distribution of protein throughout the day may also be advised.

5. Monitor Fluid Intake: Individuals with kidney disease may need to monitor their fluid intake to prevent fluid overload and electrolyte imbalances. Depending on the stage of kidney disease, fluid restrictions may be recommended to manage symptoms such as edema (swelling) and hypertension. Healthcare providers may provide guidance on the appropriate fluid intake based on individual needs and health status. Monitoring fluid intake and avoiding excessive consumption of fluids from beverages such as sodas, juices, and caffeinated drinks can help maintain fluid balance.

6. Emphasize Nutrient-Dense Foods: A kidney-friendly diet should prioritize nutrient-dense foods that provide essential vitamins, minerals, and antioxidants to support overall health and well-being. Fruits, vegetables, whole grains, lean proteins, and healthy fats should form the foundation of the diet. These foods provide essential nutrients while being lower in sodium, potassium, and phosphorus compared to processed and packaged foods. Incorporating a variety of colorful fruits and vegetables can ensure a diverse intake of vitamins, minerals, and antioxidants.

7. Individualize Based on Health Status: It's essential to individualize the kidney-friendly diet based on

factors such as the stage of kidney disease, coexisting medical conditions, medication use, nutritional status, and individual preferences. Healthcare providers, including registered dietitians, can help individuals tailor their dietary plan to meet their specific needs and goals while managing kidney disease effectively. Regular monitoring of kidney function, blood pressure, and other relevant parameters can inform dietary adjustments as needed.

8. Promote Healthy Lifestyle Habits: In addition to dietary modifications, promoting healthy lifestyle habits such as regular physical activity, smoking cessation, stress management, and adequate sleep can support overall kidney health and well-being. Physical activity can help improve cardiovascular health, maintain muscle strength, and manage weight, all of which are important for individuals with kidney disease. Stress reduction techniques such as mindfulness, meditation, and relaxation exercises can help mitigate the psychological impact of kidney disease and promote emotional well-being.

Practical Meal Planning Tips for Men Managing Kidney Disease

Meal planning is crucial for men managing kidney disease as it helps ensure a balanced and kidney-friendly diet while meeting nutritional needs and managing symptoms. Here are some practical meal planning tips tailored specifically for men with kidney disease:

1. Work with a Registered Dietitian: A registered dietitian specializing in renal nutrition can provide personalized guidance and meal plans tailored to individual nutritional needs, kidney function, and health goals. They can help optimize nutrient intake while managing restrictions on sodium, potassium, phosphorus, and protein.

2. Understand Dietary Restrictions: Familiarize yourself with the dietary restrictions associated with kidney disease, including limitations on sodium, potassium, phosphorus, and protein intake. Read food labels carefully to identify hidden sources of these nutrients and make informed choices when planning meals and snacks.

3. Plan Balanced Meals: Aim for balanced meals that include a variety of nutrient-dense foods from all food groups. Include lean proteins, such as chicken, turkey, fish, eggs, and tofu; whole grains, such as brown rice, quinoa, and whole wheat bread; plenty of fruits and vegetables; and healthy fats, such as olive oil, avocados, and nuts.

4. Portion Control: Pay attention to portion sizes to avoid overeating and to manage intake of nutrients that need to be limited, such as protein, potassium, and phosphorus. Use measuring cups, spoons, and food scales to portion out foods accurately, especially when cooking at home.

5. Limit Processed Foods: Minimize consumption of processed and packaged foods, which are often

high in sodium, phosphorus additives, and other additives that may be harmful to kidney health. Opt for fresh, whole foods whenever possible and prepare meals from scratch using simple ingredients.
6. Choose Kidney-Friendly Ingredients: Select ingredients that are low in sodium, potassium, and phosphorus to incorporate into meals and recipes. Use fresh or frozen vegetables instead of canned varieties, choose low-sodium or no-salt-added canned goods, and opt for herbs, spices, and lemon juice for flavoring instead of salt.

7. Modify Cooking Techniques: Experiment with cooking techniques that minimize the need for added salt, fat, or phosphorus additives. Try grilling, baking, steaming, roasting, or sautéing foods with minimal added oils or seasonings. Avoid breading or frying foods, as these methods can increase phosphorus and sodium content.

8. Limit High-Potassium Foods: Monitor intake of high-potassium foods, such as bananas, oranges, tomatoes, potatoes, and leafy greens, which may need to be restricted in some cases. Cook potassium-rich vegetables in water and discard the cooking liquid to reduce potassium content.

9. Use Phosphorus Binders as Directed: If prescribed phosphorus binders by your healthcare provider, take them with meals as directed to help control phosphorus absorption from food. Incorporate phosphorus binders into your meal planning

routine and take them consistently to manage phosphorus levels effectively.

10. Stay Hydrated: Drink fluids throughout the day to stay hydrated, but be mindful of fluid intake restrictions if recommended by your healthcare provider. Choose hydrating beverages such as water, herbal teas, and homemade fruit-infused water, and limit consumption of sugary drinks and caffeinated beverages.

11. Plan Ahead: Take time to plan meals and snacks in advance to ensure that you have kidney-friendly options available. Consider batch cooking and meal prepping on days when you have more time, so you have healthy meals ready to eat throughout the week.

12. Listen to Your Body: Pay attention to how different foods and meals make you feel and adjust your diet accordingly. Keep track of symptoms, such as changes in energy levels, appetite, and digestion, and discuss any concerns with your healthcare team or dietitian.

13. Seek Support: Don't hesitate to reach out for support from healthcare providers, registered dietitians, support groups, and loved ones. Managing kidney disease can be challenging, but with the right support system in place, you can navigate the journey more effectively.

PART 3: Staying Active and Fit with Kidney Disease

Debunking Exercise Myths for Men with Kidney Disease

Exercise is an important aspect of overall health and well-being for individuals with kidney disease, but there are often misconceptions or myths surrounding exercise and its safety for this population. Debunking these myths is crucial to help men with kidney disease understand the benefits of exercise and make informed decisions about incorporating physical activity into their lives. Here are some common exercise myths for men with kidney disease and the truths behind them:

- Myth: Exercise is unsafe for people with kidney disease.
- Truth: While it's essential for individuals with kidney disease to consult with their healthcare provider before starting an exercise program, regular physical activity can be safe and beneficial for most people with kidney disease. Exercise can help improve cardiovascular health, muscle

strength, flexibility, mood, and overall quality of life. However, the type, intensity, and duration of exercise should be tailored to individual health status and kidney function.

- Myth: Exercise will worsen kidney function or cause further damage to the kidneys.
- Truth: Moderate-intensity exercise is generally safe and unlikely to worsen kidney function in individuals with stable kidney disease. In fact, regular exercise may help improve cardiovascular health, blood pressure control, and insulin sensitivity, which can benefit kidney health in the long term. However, individuals with advanced kidney disease or specific complications may need to modify their exercise routine or seek guidance from a healthcare provider.

- Myth: Individuals with kidney disease should avoid strenuous or high-impact exercise.
- Truth: While certain types of high-impact or strenuous exercise may not be suitable for individuals with kidney disease, there are many safe and effective forms of physical activity that can be enjoyed. Low-impact exercises such as walking, cycling, swimming, yoga, and tai chi are generally well-tolerated and provide cardiovascular benefits without putting excessive stress on the joints or kidneys. It's important to choose activities that are appropriate for individual fitness levels and health status.

- Myth: Exercise will lead to muscle wasting or protein loss in individuals with kidney disease.
- Truth: While individuals with advanced kidney disease may experience muscle wasting or protein loss due to metabolic changes and decreased physical activity, incorporating regular exercise and resistance training can help preserve muscle mass and strength. Resistance training, such as weightlifting or bodyweight exercises, can be particularly beneficial for building muscle and improving functional capacity in individuals with kidney disease. Consulting with a healthcare provider or exercise specialist can help develop a safe and effective resistance training program.

- Myth: Individuals on dialysis should avoid exercise due to fatigue or weakness.
- Truth: While individuals on dialysis may experience fatigue or weakness, regular exercise can help improve energy levels, mood, and overall well-being. Engaging in low- to moderate-intensity exercise, such as walking, cycling, or light resistance training, can help combat fatigue, improve cardiovascular fitness, and enhance quality of life for individuals on dialysis. It's essential to listen to the body, start slowly, and gradually increase exercise intensity and duration as tolerated.

- Myth: Exercise is not necessary for individuals with kidney disease because they are already receiving medical treatment.
- Truth: Medical treatment alone may not be sufficient to address all aspects of kidney disease

and its associated complications. Regular exercise plays a critical role in supporting overall health, managing comorbidities such as hypertension and diabetes, and reducing the risk of cardiovascular disease, which is a common complication of kidney disease. Exercise can also help improve mental health, reduce stress, and enhance quality of life.

- Myth: It's too late to start exercising if you have advanced kidney disease or are on dialysis.
- Truth: It's never too late to start exercising, even for individuals with advanced kidney disease or those on dialysis. Incorporating regular physical activity into daily life can provide numerous health benefits and improve quality of life, regardless of age or stage of kidney disease. Starting with low-impact activities and gradually increasing intensity and duration as tolerated can help individuals build strength, endurance, and confidence over time.

Physical Benefits of Exercise for Kidney Health

Physical exercise offers a multitude of benefits for kidney health, supporting overall well-being and helping to manage symptoms associated with kidney disease. Here's a detailed overview of the physical benefits of exercise for kidney health:

- Improved Cardiovascular Health: Regular exercise helps improve cardiovascular fitness by strengthening the heart muscle, improving blood circulation, and lowering blood pressure. This is particularly important for individuals with kidney disease, as they are at increased risk of cardiovascular complications such as heart disease and stroke. By enhancing cardiovascular health, exercise can help reduce the risk of heart-related issues and improve overall longevity.

- Enhanced Muscle Strength and Endurance: Exercise, especially resistance training, helps build muscle strength and endurance. This is beneficial for individuals with kidney disease, as muscle wasting (sarcopenia) is a common complication, particularly in advanced stages of the disease. By engaging in regular physical activity, individuals can preserve muscle mass, improve functional capacity, and maintain independence in daily activities.

- Better Weight Management: Exercise plays a crucial role in weight management by increasing energy expenditure, promoting fat loss, and preserving lean muscle mass. Maintaining a healthy weight is important for individuals with kidney disease, as obesity and excess body fat can exacerbate complications such as hypertension, diabetes, and cardiovascular disease. Regular physical activity can help individuals achieve and maintain a healthy weight, reducing the risk of obesity-related complications.

- Improved Insulin Sensitivity: Exercise helps improve insulin sensitivity, allowing cells to better respond to insulin and regulate blood sugar levels. This is particularly beneficial for individuals with kidney disease who may have insulin resistance or diabetes, both of which are common comorbidities. By enhancing insulin sensitivity, exercise can help improve glycemic control, reduce the risk of diabetes-related complications, and support overall metabolic health.

- Enhanced Bone Health: Weight-bearing and resistance exercises help promote bone density and strength, reducing the risk of osteoporosis and bone fractures. Individuals with kidney disease are at increased risk of bone disorders such as renal osteodystrophy due to mineral imbalances and hormonal changes. By engaging in weight-bearing exercises such as walking, jogging, or dancing, individuals can help maintain bone health and reduce the risk of fractures.

- Improved Circulation and Oxygen Delivery: Exercise stimulates blood flow and circulation throughout the body, delivering oxygen and nutrients to tissues and organs, including the kidneys. Improved circulation can help support kidney function and optimize waste removal and filtration. Regular physical activity also promotes vasodilation and relaxation of blood vessels, which can help lower blood pressure and reduce the workload on the kidneys.

- Enhanced Immune Function: Regular exercise has been shown to boost immune function, reducing the risk of infections and illness. This is important for individuals with kidney disease, who may be more susceptible to infections due to compromised immune function and frequent medical interventions such as dialysis or kidney transplantation. By strengthening the immune system, exercise can help individuals better resist infections and maintain overall health.

- Reduction of Inflammation and Oxidative Stress: Chronic inflammation and oxidative stress play a role in the progression of kidney disease and the development of complications such as cardiovascular disease. Exercise has anti-inflammatory and antioxidant effects, helping to reduce inflammation and oxidative stress throughout the body. By lowering inflammation and oxidative damage, exercise can help slow the progression of kidney disease and improve overall health outcomes.

Low-Impact Exercises Tailored for Kidney Health

Low-impact exercises are particularly beneficial for individuals with kidney disease as they provide cardiovascular benefits and muscle strengthening without putting excessive stress on the joints or kidneys. These exercises can help improve overall fitness, manage symptoms, and support kidney health. Here are some low-impact exercises tailored for kidney health:

- Walking: Walking is a simple and effective low-impact exercise that can be easily incorporated into daily life. It improves cardiovascular fitness, strengthens leg muscles, and promotes overall health. Individuals with kidney disease can start with short walks and gradually increase duration and intensity as tolerated. Walking outdoors or on a treadmill allows for customization of pace and terrain.

- Cycling: Cycling is another excellent low-impact exercise that provides cardiovascular benefits and strengthens leg muscles. Riding a stationary bike or cycling outdoors allows individuals to control intensity and duration based on their fitness level. Cycling is gentle on the joints and can be adapted to individual preferences, such as leisurely rides or more intense intervals.

- Swimming and Water Aerobics: Swimming and water aerobics are ideal low-impact exercises for individuals with kidney disease, as the buoyancy of water reduces stress on the joints and provides resistance for muscle strengthening. Swimming laps, water walking, and participating in water aerobics classes can improve cardiovascular fitness, muscle tone, and flexibility. Water exercises are especially beneficial for individuals with arthritis or joint pain.

- Tai Chi and Qigong: Tai Chi and Qigong are gentle mind-body exercises that emphasize slow, flowing movements and deep breathing. These ancient practices improve balance, flexibility, and relaxation while promoting overall well-being. Tai Chi and Qigong are low-impact exercises suitable for individuals of all ages and fitness levels, making them ideal for those with kidney disease who may have mobility limitations.

- Yoga and Pilates: Yoga and Pilates are low-impact exercises that focus on strengthening the core, improving flexibility, and promoting relaxation. These mind-body practices incorporate controlled movements, breath awareness, and mindfulness techniques to enhance physical and mental well-being. Yoga and Pilates classes can be modified to accommodate individuals with kidney disease, with options for chair yoga or gentle stretches.

- Elliptical Training: Using an elliptical machine provides a low-impact cardiovascular workout that simulates walking or running without the impact on the joints. Elliptical training strengthens the lower body muscles, improves cardiovascular fitness, and burns calories effectively. Individuals with kidney disease can adjust the resistance and incline settings to customize the intensity of their workout.

- Resistance Training: Resistance training, also known as strength training or weightlifting, involves using resistance bands, free weights, or weight machines to build muscle strength and endurance. It is essential for individuals with kidney disease to incorporate resistance training into their exercise routine to combat muscle wasting (sarcopenia) and preserve functional capacity. Resistance training exercises should target major muscle groups and be performed with proper form and technique.

- Seated Exercises: Seated exercises are suitable for individuals with mobility limitations or balance issues. These exercises can be performed while sitting in a chair or wheelchair and focus on improving strength, flexibility, and range of motion. Seated exercises may include arm curls, leg lifts, shoulder rolls, and seated yoga poses. They can be adapted to individual abilities and fitness levels.

- When incorporating low-impact exercises into a fitness routine for kidney health, it's essential to start slowly and gradually increase intensity and duration as tolerated. Individuals with kidney disease should listen to their bodies, avoid overexertion, and consult with a healthcare provider before beginning any new exercise program. Working with a certified fitness trainer or physical therapist experienced in working with individuals with kidney disease can provide additional guidance and support in developing a safe and effective exercise plan

Gentle Strength Training Strategies for Men Managing Kidney Disease

Gentle strength training is a valuable component of exercise for men managing kidney disease. It helps build muscle strength, improve functional capacity, and enhance overall well-being without putting excessive stress on the body or kidneys. Here's a detailed overview of gentle strength training strategies tailored for men with kidney disease:

- Consult with Healthcare Provider: Before starting any strength training program, it's essential for men with kidney disease to consult with their healthcare provider, particularly if they have advanced kidney disease or other medical conditions. A healthcare provider can assess individual health status, provide guidance on exercise safety, and offer recommendations tailored to specific needs and goals.

- Start Slowly and Progress Gradually: When beginning a strength training program, it's important to start slowly and progress gradually to avoid injury and overexertion. Begin with light weights or resistance bands and perform a low number of repetitions and sets. As strength and endurance improve, gradually increase the weight, repetitions, and sets over time.

- Focus on Form and Technique: Proper form and technique are essential for safe and effective strength training. Pay attention to proper body alignment, posture, and movement patterns to prevent injury and maximize benefits. If unsure about proper form, consider working with a certified fitness trainer or physical therapist experienced in strength training for individuals with kidney disease.

- Choose Low-Impact Exercises: Select low-impact strength training exercises that are gentle on the joints and suitable for individuals with kidney disease. Avoid high-impact exercises or activities that place excessive stress on the body, such as heavy lifting, jumping, or vigorous plyometric movements. Instead, opt for exercises that emphasize controlled movements and gradual progression.

- Use Light Weights or Resistance Bands: Light weights or resistance bands are excellent tools for gentle strength training. They provide resistance to muscles without placing undue stress on the joints or kidneys. Start with light resistance and gradually increase as strength improves. Resistance bands are particularly versatile and can be easily adjusted to accommodate different fitness levels.

- Focus on Major Muscle Groups: Incorporate exercises that target major muscle groups throughout the body, including the chest, back, shoulders, arms, legs, and core. Choose a variety of exercises that work different muscle groups to ensure a balanced and comprehensive workout. Examples of gentle strength training exercises include bicep curls, shoulder presses, chest presses, rows, squats, and lunges.

- Perform Bodyweight Exercises: Bodyweight exercises are an excellent option for gentle strength training, as they require minimal equipment and can be performed anywhere. Examples of bodyweight exercises include push-ups, squats, lunges, planks, and leg lifts. These exercises help build strength and improve stability without the need for additional resistance.

- Incorporate Stability and Balance Exercises: Stability and balance exercises are essential for men with kidney disease, as they help improve coordination, posture, and overall stability. Include exercises that challenge balance and stability, such as single-leg stands, heel-to-toe walks, and balance board exercises. These exercises can help reduce the risk of falls and injuries, especially in older adults with kidney disease.

- Listen to Your Body: Pay attention to how your body responds to strength training and adjust your routine accordingly. If you experience pain, discomfort, or excessive fatigue, stop the exercise and consult with a healthcare provider. It's important to listen to your body's signals and avoid pushing yourself beyond your limits.

- Rest and Recovery: Allow adequate rest and recovery between strength training sessions to allow muscles to repair and grow. Aim for at least 48 hours of rest between sessions targeting the same muscle groups. Incorporate gentle stretching and relaxation techniques into your routine to promote flexibility and reduce muscle tension.

- Stay Hydrated and Nourished: Drink plenty of fluids before, during, and after strength training sessions to stay hydrated and support kidney function. Ensure adequate intake of protein and nutrients to support muscle repair and recovery. A balanced diet rich in lean protein, fruits, vegetables, whole grains, and healthy fats can help support overall health and fitness.

The Mental Health Benefits of Exercise in Kidney Disease Management

Exercise not only benefits physical health but also plays a significant role in promoting mental well-being for individuals managing kidney disease. Here's a detailed look at the mental health benefits of exercise in kidney disease management:

- Reduction of Stress and Anxiety: Regular exercise is known to reduce stress and anxiety levels by promoting the release of endorphins, also known as "feel-good" hormones, in the brain. Individuals with kidney disease often experience stress and anxiety related to the challenges of managing their condition, including medical appointments, treatments, dietary restrictions, and lifestyle changes. Engaging in physical activity provides a natural outlet for stress relief and helps promote relaxation and emotional well-being.

- Improved Mood and Emotional Health: Exercise has been shown to improve mood and emotional health by increasing levels of serotonin and dopamine, neurotransmitters associated with feelings of happiness and well-being. Men with kidney disease may experience mood fluctuations and emotional distress due to the impact of the disease on their daily lives and future outlook. Regular exercise can help lift mood, boost self-esteem, and promote a more positive outlook on life.

- Enhanced Cognitive Function: Physical activity has been linked to improved cognitive function and brain health, including memory, attention, and executive function. Engaging in regular exercise may help individuals with kidney disease maintain cognitive function and reduce the risk of cognitive decline associated with aging and chronic illness. Improved cognitive function can enhance quality of life and facilitate better management of kidney disease and related symptoms.

- Stress Management and Coping Skills: Exercise provides a healthy outlet for managing stress and coping with the challenges of living with kidney disease. By focusing on physical activity, individuals can temporarily shift their attention away from worries and concerns, allowing for a sense of relief and relaxation. Developing coping skills through exercise, such as goal-setting, problem-solving, and resilience-building, can help individuals better manage stressors and adapt to changes in their health status.

- Social Interaction and Support: Participating in group exercise classes or recreational activities provides opportunities for social interaction and support, which are essential for mental health and well-being. Building connections with others who share similar experiences can reduce feelings of isolation and loneliness commonly experienced by individuals with chronic illness. Group exercise settings also offer encouragement, motivation, and camaraderie, fostering a sense of belonging and community.

- Distraction from Symptoms and Pain: Exercise serves as a distraction from symptoms and pain associated with kidney disease, allowing individuals to focus on the present moment and engage in enjoyable activities. By shifting their attention to physical activity, individuals may experience temporary relief from discomfort and pain, as well as a sense of accomplishment and empowerment. Engaging in activities that bring joy and fulfillment can improve overall mood and quality of life.

- Improved Sleep Quality: Regular exercise has been shown to improve sleep quality and duration, which are essential for overall health and well-being. Individuals with kidney disease may experience sleep disturbances due to factors such as restless legs syndrome, frequent urination, or side effects of medications. Engaging in physical activity during the day can help regulate sleep-wake cycles, promote relaxation, and improve sleep onset and continuity.

- Empowerment and Self-Efficacy: Incorporating exercise into a daily routine empowers individuals with kidney disease to take an active role in managing their health and well-being. By setting goals, tracking progress, and achieving milestones through exercise, individuals gain a sense of control and mastery over their condition. This increased sense of self-efficacy can boost confidence, motivation, and resilience in coping with the challenges of kidney disease.

PART 4: HEALTHY AND DELICIOUS RECIPES

BREAKFAST

Vegetable Omelette

Ingredients:
2 large eggs
1/4 cup diced bell peppers
1/4 cup diced onions
1/4 cup diced tomatoes
1 tablespoon chopped fresh parsley
Salt and pepper to taste
1 teaspoon olive oil for cooking

Preparation:
In a bowl, whisk the eggs until well beaten. Stir in the diced vegetables and chopped parsley. Season with salt and pepper.
Heat olive oil in a non-stick skillet over medium heat. Pour the egg mixture into the skillet and cook until the edges are set.
Using a spatula, gently lift the edges of the omelette and tilt the skillet to allow the uncooked eggs to flow underneath.
Once the omelette is cooked through and golden brown on the bottom, fold it in half and transfer to a plate. Serve hot.

Nutritional Information (per serving):

Sodium: 200mg
Potassium: 250mg
Phosphorus: 120mg
Protein: 12g
Calories: 150

Greek Yogurt Parfait

Ingredients:
1/2 cup low-fat Greek yogurt
1/4 cup fresh berries (e.g., strawberries, blueberries, raspberries)
1 tablespoon chopped almonds or walnuts
1 teaspoon honey (optional)

Preparation:
In a serving glass or bowl, layer the Greek yogurt, fresh berries, and chopped nuts.
Drizzle with honey if desired.
Serve immediately or refrigerate until ready to eat.

Nutritional Information (per serving):
Sodium: 60mg
Potassium: 180mg
Phosphorus: 100mg
Protein: 10g
Calories: 120

Spinach and Mushroom Frittata

Ingredients:
4 large eggs
1/2 cup chopped spinach

1/4 cup sliced mushrooms
1 tablespoon grated Parmesan cheese
Salt and pepper to taste
1 teaspoon olive oil for cooking

Preparation:
Preheat the oven to 350°F (175°C).
In a bowl, whisk the eggs until well beaten. Stir in the chopped spinach, sliced mushrooms, and grated Parmesan cheese. Season with salt and pepper.
Heat olive oil in an oven-safe skillet over medium heat. Pour the egg mixture into the skillet and cook for 3-4 minutes, until the edges are set.
Transfer the skillet to the preheated oven and bake for 10-12 minutes, or until the frittata is cooked through and golden brown on top.
Remove from the oven and let cool slightly before slicing and serving.

Nutritional Information (per serving):
Sodium: 220mg
Potassium: 280mg
Phosphorus: 160mg
Protein: 14g
Calories: 180

Banana-Oat Pancakes

Ingredients:
1 ripe banana, mashed
1/4 cup old-fashioned oats
1 large egg
1/4 teaspoon ground cinnamon

1/4 teaspoon vanilla extract
1 teaspoon olive oil for cooking

Preparation:
In a bowl, combine the mashed banana, oats, egg, cinnamon, and vanilla extract until well mixed.
Heat olive oil in a non-stick skillet over medium heat. Pour the pancake batter into the skillet, using about 2 tablespoons for each pancake.
Cook for 2-3 minutes on each side, until golden brown and cooked through.
Serve warm with a drizzle of honey or a dollop of Greek yogurt if desired.

Nutritional Information (per serving):
Sodium: 80mg
Potassium: 250mg
Phosphorus: 120mg
Protein: 6g
Calories: 150

Avocado Toast with Poached Egg

Ingredients:
1 slice whole wheat bread, toasted
1/4 ripe avocado, mashed
1 large egg
Salt and pepper to taste
1 teaspoon chopped fresh cilantro or parsley

Preparation:
Spread the mashed avocado evenly on the toasted whole wheat bread. Season with salt and pepper.

Fill a small saucepan with water and bring to a simmer.
Crack the egg into a small bowl.
Gently slide the egg into the simmering water and poach for 3-4 minutes, until the whites are set but the yolk is still runny.
Using a slotted spoon, carefully remove the poached egg from the water and place it on top of the avocado toast.
Garnish with chopped cilantro or parsley before serving.

Nutritional Information (per serving):
Sodium: 150mg
Potassium: 200mg
Phosphorus: 140mg
Protein: 8g
Calories: 180

Quinoa Breakfast Bowl

Ingredients:
1/2 cup cooked quinoa
1/4 cup low-fat cottage cheese
1/4 cup diced mango or pineapple
1 tablespoon chopped almonds or walnuts
1 teaspoon honey (optional)

Preparation:
In a serving bowl, combine the cooked quinoa, low-fat cottage cheese, diced mango or pineapple, and chopped nuts.
Drizzle with honey if desired.
Serve immediately or refrigerate until ready to eat.

Nutritional Information (per serving):
Sodium: 120mg
Potassium: 200mg
Phosphorus: 150mg
Protein: 10g
Calories: 180

Egg and Vegetable Breakfast Burrito

Ingredients:
1 large whole wheat tortilla
2 large eggs, scrambled
1/4 cup diced bell peppers
1/4 cup diced onions
1/4 cup salsa (low-sodium)
1 tablespoon chopped fresh cilantro
Salt and pepper to taste

Preparation:
Heat the whole wheat tortilla in a dry skillet over medium heat until warmed through.
In a separate skillet, scramble the eggs until cooked through. Stir in the diced bell peppers and onions, and cook until tender.
Spoon the scrambled egg mixture onto the warmed tortilla. Top with salsa and chopped cilantro.
Fold the sides of the tortilla over the filling to form a burrito.
Serve warm with additional salsa on the side if desired.

Nutritional Information (per serving):
Sodium: 250mg
Potassium: 230mg

Phosphorus: 180mg
Protein: 14g
Calories: 220

Blueberry-Almond Smoothie

Ingredients:
1/2 cup frozen blueberries
1/2 banana
1/4 cup low-fat Greek yogurt
1 tablespoon almond butter
1/2 cup unsweetened almond milk
1 teaspoon honey (optional)

Preparation:
In a blender, combine the frozen blueberries, banana, Greek yogurt, almond butter, and almond milk.
Blend until smooth and creamy.
Taste and add honey if additional sweetness is desired.
Pour into a glass and serve immediately.

Nutritional Information (per serving):
Sodium: 80mg
Potassium: 250mg
Phosphorus: 120mg
Protein: 8g
Calories: 200

Cottage Cheese Pancakes

Ingredients:
1/2 cup low-fat cottage cheese
2 large eggs

2 tablespoons whole wheat flour
1/4 teaspoon baking powder
1/4 teaspoon vanilla extract
1 teaspoon olive oil for cooking
Preparation:
In a blender or food processor, combine the low-fat cottage cheese, eggs, whole wheat flour, baking powder, and vanilla extract. Blend until smooth.
Heat olive oil in a non-stick skillet over medium heat. Pour the pancake batter into the skillet, using about 2 tablespoons for each pancake.
Cook for 2-3 minutes on each side, until golden brown and cooked through.
Serve warm with fresh fruit or a drizzle of maple syrup if desired.

Nutritional Information (per serving):
Sodium: 220mg
Potassium: 180mg
Phosphorus: 160mg
Protein: 14g
Calories: 190

Apple-Cinnamon Overnight Oats

Ingredients:
1/2 cup old-fashioned oats
1/2 cup unsweetened almond milk
1/4 cup grated apple
1 tablespoon chopped almonds or walnuts
1/4 teaspoon ground cinnamon
1 teaspoon honey (optional)

Preparation:
In a mason jar or bowl, combine the old-fashioned oats, almond milk, grated apple, chopped nuts, ground cinnamon, and honey if desired.
Stir until well combined, then cover and refrigerate overnight.
In the morning, stir the oats and add a splash of almond milk if needed to achieve desired consistency.
Serve chilled or at room temperature.

Nutritional Information (per serving):
Sodium: 80mg
Potassium: 200mg
Phosphorus: 120mg
Protein: 6g
Calories: 180

LUNCH

Grilled Chicken Salad with Lemon-Tahini Dressing

Ingredients:
4 oz boneless, skinless chicken breast
2 cups mixed salad greens
1/4 cup cherry tomatoes, halved
1/4 cucumber, sliced
1 tablespoon chopped red onion
1 tablespoon chopped fresh parsley
1 tablespoon tahini
1 tablespoon lemon juice
1 teaspoon olive oil

Salt and pepper to taste

Preparation:
Season the chicken breast with salt and pepper, then grill or pan-sear until cooked through. Slice thinly.
In a large bowl, combine the mixed salad greens, cherry tomatoes, cucumber, red onion, and sliced chicken.
In a small bowl, whisk together the tahini, lemon juice, and olive oil to make the dressing.
Drizzle the dressing over the salad and toss to coat evenly. Garnish with chopped parsley before serving.

Nutritional Information (per serving):
Sodium: 220mg
Potassium: 350mg
Phosphorus: 200mg
Protein: 20g
Calories: 250

Quinoa and Black Bean Stuffed Bell Peppers

Ingredients:
2 large bell peppers, halved and seeds removed
1/2 cup cooked quinoa
1/2 cup canned black beans, rinsed and drained
1/4 cup diced tomatoes
1/4 cup diced red onion
1/4 cup shredded low-fat cheese
1 tablespoon chopped fresh cilantro
1/2 teaspoon ground cumin
Salt and pepper to taste

Preparation:
Preheat the oven to 375°F (190°C).
In a bowl, combine the cooked quinoa, black beans, diced tomatoes, red onion, shredded cheese, chopped cilantro, ground cumin, salt, and pepper.
Spoon the quinoa and black bean mixture into the halved bell peppers, dividing evenly.
Place the stuffed bell peppers in a baking dish and bake for 25-30 minutes, until the peppers are tender and the filling is heated through.
Serve hot, garnished with additional cilantro if desired.

Nutritional Information (per serving):
Sodium: 250mg
Potassium: 380mg
Phosphorus: 180mg
Protein: 12g
Calories: 230

Salmon and Asparagus Foil Packets

Ingredients:
4 oz salmon fillet
1/2 cup asparagus spears
1/4 cup diced bell peppers
1/4 cup sliced zucchini
1 tablespoon chopped fresh dill
1 tablespoon lemon juice
1 teaspoon olive oil
Salt and pepper to taste

Preparation:
Preheat the oven to 375°F (190°C).
Place a piece of aluminum foil on a baking sheet and lightly coat with non-stick cooking spray.
Place the salmon fillet in the center of the foil and arrange the asparagus, bell peppers, and zucchini around it.
Drizzle the salmon and vegetables with olive oil and lemon juice. Season with salt, pepper, and chopped dill.
Fold the edges of the foil to create a packet, sealing tightly.
Bake for 15-20 minutes, until the salmon is cooked through and the vegetables are tender.
Carefully open the foil packet and transfer the salmon and vegetables to a plate to serve.

Nutritional Information (per serving):
Sodium: 220mg
Potassium: 420mg
Phosphorus: 200mg
Protein: 20g
Calories: 250

Turkey and Vegetable Stir-Fry

Ingredients:
4 oz turkey breast, thinly sliced
1 cup mixed vegetables (e.g., bell peppers, broccoli, carrots, snap peas)
1/4 cup sliced mushrooms
2 tablespoons low-sodium soy sauce
1 tablespoon rice vinegar
1 teaspoon sesame oil
1 teaspoon minced garlic
1/2 teaspoon grated ginger

Cooked brown rice for serving

Preparation:
Heat a non-stick skillet or wok over medium-high heat. Add the sliced turkey breast and cook until browned and cooked through. Remove from the skillet and set aside.
In the same skillet, add the mixed vegetables and sliced mushrooms. Stir-fry until the vegetables are tender-crisp.
In a small bowl, whisk together the low-sodium soy sauce, rice vinegar, sesame oil, minced garlic, and grated ginger. Return the cooked turkey breast to the skillet, then pour the sauce over the turkey and vegetables. Stir to coat evenly and heat through.
Serve the turkey and vegetable stir-fry hot over cooked brown rice.

Nutritional Information (per serving):
Sodium: 280mg
Potassium: 450mg
Phosphorus: 200mg
Protein: 22g
Calories: 270

Vegetarian Lentil Soup

Ingredients:
1/2 cup dried green lentils, rinsed
2 cups low-sodium vegetable broth
1/2 cup diced carrots
1/2 cup diced celery
1/4 cup diced onion
1 clove garlic, minced
1/2 teaspoon dried thyme

1/2 teaspoon dried oregano
Salt and pepper to taste
1 tablespoon chopped fresh parsley

Preparation:
In a large pot, combine the dried green lentils, low-sodium vegetable broth, diced carrots, diced celery, diced onion, minced garlic, dried thyme, and dried oregano.
Bring the soup to a boil, then reduce the heat to low and simmer for 20-25 minutes, until the lentils and vegetables are tender.
Season the soup with salt and pepper to taste. Stir in chopped fresh parsley before serving.
Serve hot as a standalone meal or with whole wheat bread for a complete lunch.

Nutritional Information (per serving):
Sodium: 220mg
Potassium: 400mg
Phosphorus: 180mg
Protein: 14g
Calories: 220

Mediterranean Chickpea Salad

Ingredients:
1 cup canned chickpeas, rinsed and drained
1/2 cup diced cucumber
1/2 cup cherry tomatoes, halved
1/4 cup diced red onion
1/4 cup sliced Kalamata olives
2 tablespoons crumbled feta cheese
1 tablespoon chopped fresh parsley

1 tablespoon olive oil
1 tablespoon lemon juice
Salt and pepper to taste

Preparation:
In a large bowl, combine the canned chickpeas, diced cucumber, cherry tomatoes, diced red onion, sliced Kalamata olives, crumbled feta cheese, and chopped fresh parsley.
Drizzle the salad with olive oil and lemon juice. Season with salt and pepper to taste.
Toss the salad gently to coat evenly.
Serve chilled or at room temperature as a light and refreshing lunch option.

Nutritional Information (per serving):
Sodium: 280mg
Potassium: 370mg
Phosphorus: 190mg
Protein: 10g
Calories: 230

Tuna Salad Lettuce Wraps

Ingredients:
1 can (5 oz) water-packed tuna, drained
2 tablespoons plain Greek yogurt
1 tablespoon chopped celery
1 tablespoon chopped red onion
1 tablespoon chopped fresh dill or parsley
1 teaspoon lemon juice
Salt and pepper to taste
4 large lettuce leaves (e.g., butter lettuce, romaine)

Preparation:
In a bowl, combine the drained tuna, plain Greek yogurt, chopped celery, chopped red onion, chopped fresh dill or parsley, and lemon juice. Mix well.
Season the tuna salad with salt and pepper to taste.
Spoon the tuna salad onto the large lettuce leaves, dividing evenly.
Wrap the lettuce leaves around the tuna salad to form wraps.
Serve immediately as a light and protein-rich lunch option.

Nutritional Information (per serving):
Sodium: 250mg
Potassium: 280mg
Phosphorus: 220mg
Protein: 20g
Calories: 200

Eggplant and Tomato Pasta

Ingredients:
1 cup whole wheat pasta (e.g., penne, fusilli)
1 cup diced eggplant
1/2 cup diced tomatoes
1/4 cup sliced mushrooms
1 clove garlic, minced
1 tablespoon olive oil
1 tablespoon chopped fresh basil
Salt and pepper to taste
Grated Parmesan cheese for serving (optional)

Preparation:
Cook the whole wheat pasta according to package instructions until al dente. Drain and set aside.
Heat olive oil in a skillet over medium heat. Add the diced eggplant, diced tomatoes, sliced mushrooms, and minced garlic.
Sautee until the vegetables are tender and lightly browned. Add the cooked pasta to the skillet and toss to combine with the vegetables.
Season with salt and pepper to taste. Stir in chopped fresh basil.
Serve hot, garnished with grated Parmesan cheese if desired.

Nutritional Information (per serving):
Sodium: 180mg
Potassium: 320mg
Phosphorus: 150mg
Protein: 8g
Calories: 220

Vegetable and Lentil Curry

Ingredients:
1/2 cup dried red lentils, rinsed
1 cup low-sodium vegetable broth
1/2 cup diced potatoes
1/2 cup diced carrots
1/2 cup diced bell peppers
1/4 cup diced onions
1 clove garlic, minced
1 tablespoon curry powder
1 teaspoon olive oil

1 tablespoon chopped fresh cilantro
Cooked brown rice for serving

Preparation:
In a large pot, combine the dried red lentils, low-sodium vegetable broth, diced potatoes, diced carrots, diced bell peppers, diced onions, minced garlic, and curry powder.
Bring the mixture to a boil, then reduce the heat to low and simmer for 20-25 minutes, until the lentils and vegetables are tender.
Heat olive oil in a skillet over medium heat. Add the cooked lentil and vegetable mixture to the skillet and cook for an additional 5 minutes, stirring occasionally.
Serve the vegetable and lentil curry hot over cooked brown rice.
Garnish with chopped fresh cilantro before serving.

Nutritional Information (per serving):
Sodium: 220mg
Potassium: 380mg
Phosphorus: 200mg
Protein: 12g
Calories: 240

Turkey and Avocado Wrap

Ingredients:
2 oz sliced turkey breast
1/4 avocado, mashed
1 whole wheat tortilla
1/4 cup shredded lettuce
1/4 cup sliced cucumber
1 tablespoon hummus (optional)

Salt and pepper to taste

Preparation:
Spread the mashed avocado evenly on the whole wheat tortilla. Season with salt and pepper.
Layer the sliced turkey breast, shredded lettuce, and sliced cucumber on top of the mashed avocado.
Optional: spread a thin layer of hummus on the tortilla before adding the other ingredients for extra flavor.
Roll up the tortilla tightly to form a wrap.
Slice the wrap in half diagonally and serve immediately.

Nutritional Information (per serving):
Sodium: 250mg
Potassium: 300mg
Phosphorus: 200mg
Protein: 14g
Calories: 220

DINNER

Grilled Lemon Herb Chicken

Ingredients:
4 oz boneless, skinless chicken breast
1 tablespoon olive oil
1 tablespoon fresh lemon juice
1 teaspoon minced garlic
1 teaspoon chopped fresh rosemary
Salt and pepper to taste

Preparation:
In a small bowl, whisk together the olive oil, lemon juice, minced garlic, chopped rosemary, salt, and pepper to make the marinade.
Place the chicken breast in a shallow dish and pour the marinade over it, turning to coat evenly. Cover and refrigerate for at least 30 minutes.
Preheat the grill to medium-high heat. Remove the chicken from the marinade and discard any excess marinade.
Grill the chicken breast for 6-8 minutes per side, or until cooked through and no longer pink in the center.
Serve hot, garnished with additional chopped fresh herbs if desired.

Nutritional Information (per serving):
Sodium: 180mg
Potassium: 280mg
Phosphorus: 200mg
Protein: 25g
Calories: 220

Baked Salmon with Roasted Vegetables

Ingredients:
4 oz salmon fillet
1/2 cup diced sweet potatoes
1/2 cup diced zucchini
1/2 cup diced bell peppers
1/4 cup sliced red onion
1 tablespoon olive oil
1 teaspoon dried thyme
Salt and pepper to taste

Preparation:
Preheat the oven to 400°F (200°C). Line a baking sheet with parchment paper.
Place the diced sweet potatoes, zucchini, bell peppers, and red onion on the prepared baking sheet. Drizzle with olive oil and sprinkle with dried thyme, salt, and pepper. Toss to coat evenly.
Bake in the preheated oven for 20-25 minutes, stirring halfway through, until the vegetables are tender and lightly browned.
Season the salmon fillet with salt and pepper. Place it on the baking sheet with the roasted vegetables.
Bake for an additional 12-15 minutes, or until the salmon is cooked through and flakes easily with a fork.
Serve hot, accompanied by the roasted vegetables.

Nutritional Information (per serving):
Sodium: 200mg
Potassium: 550mg
Phosphorus: 220mg
Protein: 22g
Calories: 280

Turkey and Vegetable Stir-Fry

Ingredients:
4 oz turkey breast, thinly sliced
1 cup mixed vegetables (e.g., bell peppers, broccoli, carrots, snap peas)
1/4 cup sliced mushrooms
2 tablespoons low-sodium soy sauce
1 tablespoon rice vinegar
1 teaspoon sesame oil

1 teaspoon minced garlic
1/2 teaspoon grated ginger
Cooked brown rice for serving

Preparation:
Heat a non-stick skillet or wok over medium-high heat. Add the sliced turkey breast and cook until browned and cooked through. Remove from the skillet and set aside.
In the same skillet, add the mixed vegetables and sliced mushrooms. Stir-fry until the vegetables are tender-crisp.
In a small bowl, whisk together the low-sodium soy sauce, rice vinegar, sesame oil, minced garlic, and grated ginger. Return the cooked turkey breast to the skillet, then pour the sauce over the turkey and vegetables. Stir to coat evenly and heat through.
Serve the turkey and vegetable stir-fry hot over cooked brown rice.

Nutritional Information (per serving):
Sodium: 280mg
Potassium: 450mg
Phosphorus: 200mg
Protein: 22g
Calories: 270

Vegetarian Chickpea and Spinach Curry

Ingredients:
1 cup cooked chickpeas
2 cups fresh spinach leaves
1/2 cup diced tomatoes
1/4 cup diced onions
1/4 cup canned coconut milk (light)

1 tablespoon olive oil
1 teaspoon curry powder
1/2 teaspoon minced garlic
Salt and pepper to taste

Preparation:
Heat olive oil in a skillet over medium heat. Add the diced onions and minced garlic, and sauté until softened.
Stir in the curry powder and cook for another minute until fragrant.
Add the diced tomatoes and cooked chickpeas to the skillet. Cook for 5 minutes, allowing the flavors to meld.
Pour in the canned coconut milk and bring the mixture to a simmer.
Add the fresh spinach leaves to the skillet and cook until wilted.
Season with salt and pepper to taste.
Serve hot, accompanied by cooked brown rice or whole wheat naan bread if desired.

Nutritional Information (per serving):
Sodium: 180mg
Potassium: 380mg
Phosphorus: 160mg
Protein: 12g
Calories: 220

Lemon Garlic Shrimp Pasta

Ingredients:
2 oz whole wheat spaghetti
4 oz shrimp, peeled and deveined
1 tablespoon olive oil

1 teaspoon minced garlic
1 tablespoon fresh lemon juice
1/4 teaspoon lemon zest
1 tablespoon chopped fresh parsley
Salt and pepper to taste

Preparation:
Cook the whole wheat spaghetti according to package instructions until al dente. Drain and set aside.
Heat olive oil in a skillet over medium heat. Add the minced garlic and cook until fragrant.
Add the shrimp to the skillet and cook for 2-3 minutes on each side, until pink and opaque.
Stir in the cooked spaghetti, fresh lemon juice, lemon zest, and chopped parsley. Toss to combine and heat through.
Season with salt and pepper to taste.
Serve hot, garnished with additional chopped parsley if desired.

Nutritional Information (per serving):
Sodium: 200mg
Potassium: 220mg
Phosphorus: 180mg
Protein: 20g
Calories: 250

Turkey Meatball and Vegetable Skewers

Ingredients:
4 oz lean ground turkey
1/4 cup whole wheat breadcrumbs
1/4 cup grated Parmesan cheese
1/4 cup diced bell peppers

1/4 cup diced zucchini
1/4 cup diced red onion
1 tablespoon chopped fresh parsley
1 teaspoon minced garlic
Salt and pepper to taste
Wooden skewers, soaked in water

Preparation:
In a bowl, combine the lean ground turkey, whole wheat breadcrumbs, grated Parmesan cheese, diced bell peppers, diced zucchini, diced red onion, chopped fresh parsley, minced garlic, salt, and pepper.
Mix until well combined, then shape the mixture into small meatballs.
Thread the turkey meatballs onto the soaked wooden skewers, alternating with the diced vegetables.
Preheat a grill or grill pan over medium heat. Lightly coat with non-stick cooking spray.
Grill the skewers for 8-10 minutes, turning occasionally, until the turkey meatballs are cooked through and the vegetables are tender.
Serve hot, accompanied by cooked quinoa or brown rice if desired.

Nutritional Information (per serving):
Sodium: 240mg
Potassium: 280mg
Phosphorus: 220mg
Protein: 18g
Calories: 240

Eggplant Parmesan

Ingredients:
1 medium eggplant, sliced into rounds
1/2 cup whole wheat breadcrumbs
1/4 cup grated Parmesan cheese
1/4 cup marinara sauce (low-sodium)
1/4 cup shredded part-skim mozzarella cheese
1 tablespoon olive oil
1/2 teaspoon dried oregano
Salt and pepper to taste

Preparation:
Preheat the oven to 400°F (200°C). Line a baking sheet with parchment paper.
In a shallow dish, combine the whole wheat breadcrumbs, grated Parmesan cheese, dried oregano, salt, and pepper.
Dip each eggplant slice into the breadcrumb mixture, coating both sides evenly.
Place the coated eggplant slices on the prepared baking sheet. Drizzle with olive oil.
Bake in the preheated oven for 20-25 minutes, flipping halfway through, until the eggplant is tender and golden brown.
Remove the baking sheet from the oven and spoon marinara sauce over each eggplant slice. Top with shredded mozzarella cheese.
Return to the oven and bake for an additional 5-7 minutes, or until the cheese is melted and bubbly.
Serve hot, garnished with chopped fresh basil if desired.

Nutritional Information (per serving):
Sodium: 200mg
Potassium: 320mg

Phosphorus: 180mg
Protein: 10g
Calories: 210

Vegetable and Tofu Stir-Fry

Ingredients:
4 oz firm tofu, cubed
1 cup mixed vegetables (e.g., bell peppers, broccoli, carrots, snap peas)
1/4 cup sliced mushrooms
2 tablespoons low-sodium soy sauce
1 tablespoon rice vinegar
1 teaspoon sesame oil
1 teaspoon minced garlic
1/2 teaspoon grated ginger
Cooked brown rice for serving

Preparation:
Heat a non-stick skillet or wok over medium-high heat. Add the cubed tofu and cook until lightly browned on all sides. Remove from the skillet and set aside.
In the same skillet, add the mixed vegetables and sliced mushrooms. Stir-fry until the vegetables are tender-crisp.
In a small bowl, whisk together the low-sodium soy sauce, rice vinegar, sesame oil, minced garlic, and grated ginger. Return the cooked tofu to the skillet, then pour the sauce over the tofu and vegetables. Stir to coat evenly and heat through.
Serve the tofu and vegetable stir-fry hot over cooked brown rice.

Nutritional Information (per serving):
Sodium: 280mg
Potassium: 420mg
Phosphorus: 200mg
Protein: 16g
Calories: 250

Lemon Herb Baked Cod

Ingredients:
4 oz cod fillet
1 tablespoon olive oil
1 tablespoon fresh lemon juice
1 teaspoon minced garlic
1 teaspoon chopped fresh parsley
Salt and pepper to taste

Preparation:
Preheat the oven to 400°F (200°C). Line a baking sheet with parchment paper.
Place the cod fillet on the prepared baking sheet.
In a small bowl, whisk together the olive oil, lemon juice, minced garlic, chopped parsley, salt, and pepper.
Pour the lemon herb mixture over the cod fillet, spreading it evenly.
Bake in the preheated oven for 12-15 minutes, or until the cod is opaque and flakes easily with a fork.
Serve hot, garnished with additional chopped parsley and lemon wedges if desired.

Nutritional Information (per serving):
Sodium: 180mg
Potassium: 320mg
Phosphorus: 180mg

Protein: 20g
Calories: 220

Mushroom and Spinach Quinoa Risotto

Ingredients:
1/2 cup quinoa, rinsed
1 cup low-sodium vegetable broth
1/2 cup sliced mushrooms
1 cup fresh spinach leaves
1/4 cup diced onions
1 clove garlic, minced
1 tablespoon olive oil
1 tablespoon grated Parmesan cheese
Salt and pepper to taste

Preparation:
In a saucepan, bring the low-sodium vegetable broth to a simmer.
Heat olive oil in a separate skillet over medium heat. Add the diced onions and minced garlic, and sauté until softened.
Stir in the sliced mushrooms and cook until tender.
Add the rinsed quinoa to the skillet and toast for 2-3 minutes, stirring constantly.
Gradually add the simmering vegetable broth to the skillet, 1/2 cup at a time, stirring frequently and allowing the quinoa to absorb the liquid before adding more.
Once all the broth has been absorbed and the quinoa is tender, stir in the fresh spinach leaves until wilted.
Season with salt and pepper to taste. Stir in grated Parmesan cheese.
Serve hot as a satisfying and nutritious dinner option.

Nutritional Information (per serving):
Sodium: 200mg
Potassium: 320mg
Phosphorus: 180mg
Protein: 10g
Calories: 230

DESSERT

Fruit Salad with Honey-Lime Dressing

Ingredients:
1 cup diced mixed fruits (e.g., strawberries, pineapple, grapes, kiwi)
1 tablespoon honey
1 tablespoon fresh lime juice
1 teaspoon lime zest
Fresh mint leaves for garnish (optional)

Preparation:
In a bowl, combine the diced mixed fruits.
In a small bowl, whisk together the honey, fresh lime juice, and lime zest to make the dressing.
Pour the dressing over the mixed fruits and toss to coat evenly.
Garnish with fresh mint leaves if desired.
Serve chilled as a refreshing and naturally sweet dessert option.

Nutritional Information (per serving):
Sodium: 5mg
Potassium: 200mg
Phosphorus: 20mg
Protein: 1g
Calories: 70

Baked Apples with Cinnamon and Walnuts

Ingredients:
2 apples, cored and halved
1 tablespoon chopped walnuts
1/2 teaspoon ground cinnamon
1 teaspoon honey (optional)
Non-stick cooking spray

Preparation:
Preheat the oven to 375°F (190°C). Lightly coat a baking dish with non-stick cooking spray.
Place the apple halves, cut side up, in the prepared baking dish.
In a small bowl, combine the chopped walnuts and ground cinnamon.
Sprinkle the cinnamon-walnut mixture evenly over the apple halves.
Drizzle honey over the apples if desired.
Bake in the preheated oven for 20-25 minutes, or until the apples are tender and lightly browned.
Serve warm as a comforting and nutritious dessert option.

Nutritional Information (per serving):
Sodium: 0mg
Potassium: 150mg
Phosphorus: 10mg

Protein: 1g
Calories: 80

Mixed Berry Parfait

Ingredients:
1/2 cup mixed berries (e.g., strawberries, blueberries, raspberries)
1/2 cup low-fat plain Greek yogurt
2 tablespoons granola (low-sodium)
Fresh mint leaves for garnish (optional)

Preparation:
In a glass or serving dish, layer the mixed berries and low-fat plain Greek yogurt.
Repeat the layers until all ingredients are used, ending with a layer of yogurt on top.
Sprinkle granola over the top layer of yogurt.
Garnish with fresh mint leaves if desired.
Serve chilled as a light and protein-rich dessert option.

Nutritional Information (per serving):
Sodium: 30mg
Potassium: 150mg
Phosphorus: 60mg
Protein: 8g
Calories: 120

Banana-Oat Cookies

Ingredients:
2 ripe bananas, mashed
1 cup rolled oats
1/4 cup chopped nuts (e.g., almonds, walnuts)
1/4 cup raisins or dried cranberries (optional)
1 teaspoon ground cinnamon
1/2 teaspoon vanilla extract

Preparation:
Preheat the oven to 350°F (175°C). Line a baking sheet with parchment paper.
In a bowl, combine the mashed bananas, rolled oats, chopped nuts, raisins or dried cranberries (if using), ground cinnamon, and vanilla extract.
Mix until well combined.
Drop spoonfuls of the cookie dough onto the prepared baking sheet, spacing them evenly apart.
Flatten each cookie slightly with the back of a spoon.
Bake in the preheated oven for 15-18 minutes, or until the cookies are golden brown.
Allow the cookies to cool on the baking sheet for a few minutes before transferring to a wire rack to cool completely.
Serve at room temperature as a wholesome and fiber-rich dessert option.

Nutritional Information (per serving, 2 cookies):
Sodium: 0mg
Potassium: 180mg
Phosphorus: 50mg
Protein: 3g
Calories: 120

Chia Seed Pudding

Ingredients:
2 tablespoons chia seeds
1/2 cup unsweetened almond milk
1/2 teaspoon vanilla extract
1 teaspoon honey or maple syrup (optional)
Fresh berries for garnish (optional)

Preparation:
In a bowl, combine the chia seeds, unsweetened almond milk, vanilla extract, and honey or maple syrup (if using). Stir well to combine.
Cover and refrigerate for at least 2 hours or overnight, until the chia seeds have absorbed the liquid and thickened to a pudding-like consistency.
Stir the chia seed pudding before serving to redistribute the seeds.
Garnish with fresh berries if desired.
Serve chilled as a nutrient-rich and satisfying dessert option.

Nutritional Information (per serving):
Sodium: 60mg
Potassium: 100mg
Phosphorus: 80mg
Protein: 3g
Calories: 90

Peach and Yogurt Popsicles

Ingredients:
1 cup diced peaches (fresh or frozen)
1 cup low-fat plain Greek yogurt
1 tablespoon honey (optional)

Preparation:
In a blender, combine the diced peaches, low-fat plain Greek yogurt, and honey (if using).
Blend until smooth and creamy.
Pour the mixture into popsicle molds.
Insert popsicle sticks into the molds.
Freeze for at least 4 hours or until completely frozen.
To unmold the popsicles, run warm water over the outside of the molds for a few seconds.
Serve immediately as a refreshing and calcium-rich dessert option.

Nutritional Information (per serving):
Sodium: 25mg
Potassium: 180mg
Phosphorus: 70mg
Protein: 6g
Calories: 80

Frozen Yogurt Bark

Ingredients:
1 cup low-fat plain Greek yogurt
1/2 cup mixed berries (e.g., strawberries, blueberries, raspberries)
2 tablespoons chopped nuts (e.g., almonds, walnuts)

1 tablespoon honey or maple syrup (optional)

Preparation:
Line a baking sheet with parchment paper.
Spread the low-fat plain Greek yogurt evenly onto the parchment paper, forming a thin layer.
Sprinkle the mixed berries and chopped nuts over the yogurt layer.
Drizzle honey or maple syrup over the top if desired.
Place the baking sheet in the freezer and freeze for at least 2 hours, or until firm.
Once frozen, break the yogurt bark into pieces.
Serve immediately as a cool and creamy dessert option.

Nutritional Information (per serving):
Sodium: 40mg
Potassium: 150mg
Phosphorus: 70mg
Protein: 5g
Calories: 90

Coconut Chia Seed Pudding

Ingredients:
2 tablespoons chia seeds
1/2 cup coconut milk
1/2 teaspoon vanilla extract
1 teaspoon honey or maple syrup (optional)
Unsweetened shredded coconut for garnish (optional)

Preparation:
In a bowl, combine the chia seeds, coconut milk, vanilla extract, and honey or maple syrup (if using).

Stir well to combine.
Cover and refrigerate for at least 2 hours or overnight, until the chia seeds have absorbed the liquid and thickened to a pudding-like consistency.
Stir the chia seed pudding before serving to redistribute the seeds.
Garnish with unsweetened shredded coconut if desired.
Serve chilled as a creamy and tropical-inspired dessert option.

Nutritional Information (per serving):
Sodium: 10mg
Potassium: 90mg
Phosphorus: 60mg
Protein: 3g
Calories: 100

Chocolate Banana Smoothie

Ingredients:
1 ripe banana
1 tablespoon unsweetened cocoa powder
1 cup unsweetened almond milk
1/2 cup low-fat plain Greek yogurt
1 teaspoon honey or maple syrup (optional)
Ice cubes

Preparation:
In a blender, combine the ripe banana, unsweetened cocoa powder, unsweetened almond milk, low-fat plain Greek yogurt, and honey or maple syrup (if using).
Add a few ice cubes to the blender for a chilled and creamy texture.

Blend until smooth and creamy.
Pour the smoothie into glasses.
Serve immediately as a satisfying and chocolatey dessert option.

Nutritional Information (per serving):
Sodium: 60mg
Potassium: 300mg
Phosphorus: 150mg
Protein: 7g
Calories: 120

Baked Pears with Cinnamon and Almonds

Ingredients:
2 ripe pears, halved and cored
2 tablespoons chopped almonds
1/2 teaspoon ground cinnamon
1 teaspoon honey (optional)
Non-stick cooking spray

Preparation:
Preheat the oven to 375°F (190°C). Lightly coat a baking dish with non-stick cooking spray.
Place the pear halves, cut side up, in the prepared baking dish.
In a small bowl, combine the chopped almonds and ground cinnamon.
Sprinkle the cinnamon-almond mixture evenly over the pear halves.
Drizzle honey over the pears if desired.
Bake in the preheated oven for 20-25 minutes, or until the pears are tender and lightly browned.

Serve warm as a comforting and naturally sweet dessert option.

Nutritional Information (per serving):
Sodium: 0mg
Potassium: 200mg
Phosphorus: 20mg
Protein: 2g
Calories: 90

SNACKS

Greek Yogurt and Berry Parfait

Ingredients:
1/2 cup low-fat plain Greek yogurt
1/4 cup mixed berries (e.g., strawberries, blueberries, raspberries)
1 tablespoon chopped nuts (e.g., almonds, walnuts)
1 teaspoon honey or maple syrup (optional)

Preparation:
In a serving dish, layer the low-fat plain Greek yogurt, mixed berries, and chopped nuts.
Drizzle with honey or maple syrup if desired.
Serve immediately as a protein-rich and satisfying snack option.

Nutritional Information (per serving):
Sodium: 50mg
Potassium: 150mg
Phosphorus: 80mg

Protein: 8g
Calories: 100

Cucumber and Hummus Slices

Ingredients:
1 small cucumber, sliced
2 tablespoons hummus (low-sodium)

Preparation:
Arrange the cucumber slices on a plate.
Place a dollop of hummus on each cucumber slice.
Serve immediately as a refreshing and fiber-rich snack option.

Nutritional Information (per serving):
Sodium: 50mg
Potassium: 150mg
Phosphorus: 30mg
Protein: 2g
Calories: 50

Apple Slices with Almond Butter

Ingredients:
1 apple, sliced
1 tablespoon almond butter

Preparation:
Dip each apple slice into almond butter.
Serve immediately as a crunchy and nutrient-rich snack option.

Nutritional Information (per serving):
Sodium: 0mg
Potassium: 100mg
Phosphorus: 50mg
Protein: 2g
Calories: 70

Carrot Sticks with Cottage Cheese Dip

Ingredients:
1 medium carrot, cut into sticks
1/4 cup low-fat cottage cheese

Preparation:
Place the low-fat cottage cheese in a small bowl.
Serve the carrot sticks alongside the cottage cheese dip.
Serve immediately as a crunchy and protein-packed snack option.

Nutritional Information (per serving):
Sodium: 100mg
Potassium: 200mg
Phosphorus: 80mg
Protein: 5g
Calories: 50

Whole Grain Crackers with Tuna Salad

Ingredients:
4 whole grain crackers (low-sodium)
2 oz canned tuna, drained
1 tablespoon plain Greek yogurt
1 teaspoon Dijon mustard
Salt and pepper to taste

Preparation:
In a bowl, mix together the canned tuna, plain Greek yogurt, Dijon mustard, salt, and pepper.
Spread the tuna salad onto each whole grain cracker.
Serve immediately as a satisfying and protein-rich snack option.

Nutritional Information (per serving):
Sodium: 150mg
Potassium: 200mg
Phosphorus: 100mg
Protein: 10g
Calories: 100

Edamame

Ingredients:
1/2 cup cooked edamame (shelled)

Preparation:
Steam or boil the edamame until tender.
Drain and rinse under cold water.

Serve immediately as a protein-packed and fiber-rich snack option.

Nutritional Information (per serving):
Sodium: 5mg
Potassium: 100mg
Phosphorus: 50mg
Protein: 8g
Calories: 60

Yogurt-Covered Pretzels

Ingredients:
1/4 cup low-fat yogurt-covered pretzels

Preparation:
Portion out the low-fat yogurt-covered pretzels.
Serve immediately as a crunchy and slightly sweet snack option.

Nutritional Information (per serving):
Sodium: 60mg
Potassium: 30mg
Phosphorus: 30mg
Protein: 1g
Calories: 60

Banana-Oat Energy Bites

Ingredients:
1 ripe banana, mashed
1/2 cup rolled oats

2 tablespoons chopped nuts (e.g., almonds, walnuts)
1 tablespoon honey or maple syrup (optional)
1/2 teaspoon ground cinnamon

Preparation:
In a bowl, combine the mashed banana, rolled oats, chopped nuts, honey or maple syrup (if using), and ground cinnamon.
Mix until well combined.
Roll the mixture into small balls.
Serve immediately as a portable and energy-boosting snack option.

Nutritional Information (per serving, 2 energy bites):
Sodium: 0mg
Potassium: 100mg
Phosphorus: 40mg
Protein: 2g
Calories: 80

Roasted Chickpeas

Ingredients:
1/2 cup cooked chickpeas (drained and rinsed)
1 teaspoon olive oil
1/2 teaspoon ground cumin
1/2 teaspoon smoked paprika
Salt to taste

Preparation:
Preheat the oven to 400°F (200°C).
In a bowl, toss the cooked chickpeas with olive oil, ground cumin, smoked paprika, and salt until evenly coated.

Spread the chickpeas in a single layer on a baking sheet lined with parchment paper.
Roast in the preheated oven for 20-25 minutes, or until golden and crispy.
Serve immediately as a crunchy and fiber-rich snack option.

Nutritional Information (per serving):
Sodium: 50mg
Potassium: 150mg
Phosphorus: 60mg
Protein: 4g
Calories: 70

Vegetable Sushi Rolls

Ingredients:
2 nori seaweed sheets
1/2 cup cooked sushi rice
Assorted thinly sliced vegetables (e.g., cucumber, avocado, carrot)
Low-sodium soy sauce for dipping

Preparation:
Place a nori seaweed sheet on a clean surface.
Spread a layer of cooked sushi rice evenly over the nori seaweed sheet.
Arrange thinly sliced vegetables in the center of the rice.
Roll up the nori seaweed sheet tightly, enclosing the vegetables.
Repeat with the remaining nori seaweed sheet and ingredients.
Slice each sushi roll into bite-sized pieces.

Serve with low-sodium soy sauce for dipping as a flavorful and nutritious snack option.

Nutritional Information (per serving, 1 roll):
Sodium: 100mg
Potassium: 150mg
Phosphorus: 40mg
Protein: 2g
Calories: 80

SMOOTHIES

Berry Blast Smoothie

Ingredients:
1/2 cup mixed berries (e.g., strawberries, blueberries, raspberries)
1/2 ripe banana
1/2 cup low-fat plain Greek yogurt
1/2 cup unsweetened almond milk
1 tablespoon honey or maple syrup (optional)
Ice cubes

Preparation:
In a blender, combine the mixed berries, ripe banana, low-fat plain Greek yogurt, unsweetened almond milk, and honey or maple syrup (if using).
Add a few ice cubes to the blender for a chilled and creamy texture.
Blend until smooth and creamy.
Pour the smoothie into glasses.
Serve immediately as a refreshing and antioxidant-rich snack option.

Nutritional Information (per serving):
Sodium: 60mg
Potassium: 250mg
Phosphorus: 100mg
Protein: 8g
Calories: 120

Green Power Smoothie

Ingredients:
1 cup spinach leaves
1/2 ripe avocado
1/2 cup chopped cucumber
1/2 cup unsweetened almond milk
1/4 cup low-fat plain Greek yogurt
1 tablespoon fresh lemon juice
1 teaspoon honey or maple syrup (optional)
Ice cubes

Preparation:
In a blender, combine the spinach leaves, ripe avocado, chopped cucumber, unsweetened almond milk, low-fat plain Greek yogurt, fresh lemon juice, and honey or maple syrup (if using).
Add a few ice cubes to the blender for a chilled and creamy texture.
Blend until smooth and creamy.
Pour the smoothie into glasses.
Serve immediately as a nutrient-packed and energizing snack option.

Nutritional Information (per serving):

Sodium: 70mg
Potassium: 400mg
Phosphorus: 120mg
Protein: 6g
Calories: 150

Banana Almond Smoothie

Ingredients:
1 ripe banana
2 tablespoons almond butter
1/2 cup low-fat plain Greek yogurt
1/2 cup unsweetened almond milk
1 tablespoon honey or maple syrup (optional)
Ice cubes

Preparation:
In a blender, combine the ripe banana, almond butter, low-fat plain Greek yogurt, unsweetened almond milk, and honey or maple syrup (if using).
Add a few ice cubes to the blender for a chilled and creamy texture.
Blend until smooth and creamy.
Pour the smoothie into glasses.
Serve immediately as a protein-rich and satisfying snack option.

Nutritional Information (per serving):
Sodium: 70mg
Potassium: 320mg
Phosphorus: 120mg
Protein: 8g
Calories: 180

Tropical Paradise Smoothie

Ingredients:
1/2 cup diced pineapple
1/2 cup diced mango
1/2 ripe banana
1/2 cup low-fat plain Greek yogurt
1/2 cup unsweetened coconut milk
1 tablespoon shredded coconut (unsweetened)
Ice cubes

Preparation:
In a blender, combine the diced pineapple, diced mango, ripe banana, low-fat plain Greek yogurt, unsweetened coconut milk, and shredded coconut.
Add a few ice cubes to the blender for a chilled and creamy texture.
Blend until smooth and creamy.
Pour the smoothie into glasses.
Serve immediately as a tropical-inspired and vitamin-rich snack option.

Nutritional Information (per serving):
Sodium: 40mg
Potassium: 350mg
Phosphorus: 110mg
Protein: 7g
Calories: 150

Peanut Butter Banana Smoothie

Ingredients:
1 ripe banana
2 tablespoons peanut butter (unsweetened)
1/2 cup low-fat plain Greek yogurt
1/2 cup unsweetened almond milk
1 tablespoon honey or maple syrup (optional)
Ice cubes

Preparation:
In a blender, combine the ripe banana, peanut butter, low-fat plain Greek yogurt, unsweetened almond milk, and honey or maple syrup (if using).
Add a few ice cubes to the blender for a chilled and creamy texture.
Blend until smooth and creamy.
Pour the smoothie into glasses.
Serve immediately as a protein-packed and indulgent snack option.

Nutritional Information (per serving):
Sodium: 90mg
Potassium: 300mg
Phosphorus: 120mg
Protein: 9g
Calories: 200

Cherry Vanilla Smoothie

Ingredients:
1/2 cup pitted cherries (fresh or frozen)
1/2 cup low-fat plain Greek yogurt
1/2 cup unsweetened almond milk
1/2 teaspoon vanilla extract
1 tablespoon honey or maple syrup (optional)
Ice cubes

Preparation:
In a blender, combine the pitted cherries, low-fat plain Greek yogurt, unsweetened almond milk, vanilla extract, and honey or maple syrup (if using).
Add a few ice cubes to the blender for a chilled and creamy texture.
Blend until smooth and creamy.
Pour the smoothie into glasses.
Serve immediately as a refreshing and antioxidant-rich snack option.

Nutritional Information (per serving):
Sodium: 60mg
Potassium: 250mg
Phosphorus: 110mg
Protein: 7g
Calories: 140

Peach Raspberry Smoothie

Ingredients:
1/2 cup diced peaches (fresh or frozen)
1/2 cup raspberries (fresh or frozen)
1/2 cup low-fat plain Greek yogurt
1/2 cup unsweetened almond milk
1 tablespoon honey or maple syrup (optional)
Ice cubes

Preparation:
In a blender, combine the diced peaches, raspberries, low-fat plain Greek yogurt, unsweetened almond milk, and honey or maple syrup (if using).
Add a few ice cubes to the blender for a chilled and creamy texture.
Blend until smooth and creamy.
Pour the smoothie into glasses.
Serve immediately as a vitamin-packed and delicious snack option.

Nutritional Information (per serving):
Sodium: 50mg
Potassium: 270mg
Phosphorus: 110mg
Protein: 7g
Calories: 140

Chocolate Banana Protein Smoothie

Ingredients:
1 ripe banana
1 tablespoon unsweetened cocoa powder
1/2 cup low-fat plain Greek yogurt
1/2 cup unsweetened almond milk
1 tablespoon honey or maple syrup (optional)
Ice cubes

Preparation:
In a blender, combine the ripe banana, unsweetened cocoa powder, low-fat plain Greek yogurt, unsweetened almond milk, and honey or maple syrup (if using).
Add a few ice cubes to the blender for a chilled and creamy texture.
Blend until smooth and creamy.
Pour the smoothie into glasses.
Serve immediately as a protein-rich and chocolatey snack option.

Nutritional Information (per serving):
Sodium: 70mg
Potassium: 310mg
Phosphorus: 120mg
Protein: 8g
Calories: 150

Minty Pineapple Smoothie

Ingredients:
1/2 cup diced pineapple
1/2 cup low-fat plain Greek yogurt
1/2 cup unsweetened coconut milk
1 tablespoon fresh mint leaves
1 tablespoon honey or maple syrup (optional)
Ice cubes

Preparation:
In a blender, combine the diced pineapple, low-fat plain Greek yogurt, unsweetened coconut milk, fresh mint leaves, and honey or maple syrup (if using).
Add a few ice cubes to the blender for a chilled and creamy texture.
Blend until smooth and creamy.
Pour the smoothie into glasses.
Serve immediately as a tropical-inspired and refreshing snack option.

Nutritional Information (per serving):
Sodium: 60mg
Potassium: 300mg
Phosphorus: 120mg
Protein: 7g
Calories: 140

Coconut Banana Smoothie

Ingredients:
1 ripe banana
1/2 cup unsweetened coconut milk
1/2 cup low-fat plain Greek yogurt
1 tablespoon shredded coconut (unsweetened)
1 tablespoon honey or maple syrup (optional)
Ice cubes

Preparation:
In a blender, combine the ripe banana, unsweetened coconut milk, low-fat plain Greek yogurt, shredded coconut, and honey or maple syrup (if using).
Add a few ice cubes to the blender for a chilled and creamy texture.
Blend until smooth and creamy.
Pour the smoothie into glasses.
Serve immediately as a tropical-inspired and indulgent snack option.

Nutritional Information (per serving):
Sodium: 50mg
Potassium: 280mg
Phosphorus: 110mg
Protein: 7g
Calories: 150

BONUS

Shopping list

Proteins:
1. Skinless chicken breasts
2. Lean ground turkey
3. Lean cuts of beef (e.g., sirloin, tenderloin)
4. Fish (e.g., salmon, trout, tuna)
5. Shellfish (e.g., shrimp, crab)
6. Eggs
7. Low-fat plain Greek yogurt
8. Low-fat cottage cheese
9. Tofu or tempeh
10. Canned tuna or salmon (in water, low-sodium)

Vegetables:
1. Spinach
2. Kale
3. Broccoli
4. Cauliflower
5. Bell peppers (various colors)
6. Carrots
7. Zucchini
8. Cucumber
9. Tomatoes
10. Green beans

Fruits:
1. Apples
2. Bananas
3. Berries (e.g., strawberries, blueberries, raspberries)

4. Oranges
5. Grapes
6. Pineapple
7. Mango
8. Peaches
9. Kiwi
10. Pears

Grains and Starches:
Brown rice
1. Quinoa
2. Whole grain pasta
3. Whole grain bread (low-sodium)
4. Oats
5. Barley
6. Bulgur
7. Whole wheat tortillas
8. Sweet potatoes
9. White potatoes

Dairy and Dairy Alternatives:
1. Unsweetened almond milk
2. Unsweetened coconut milk
3. Low-fat cheese (e.g., mozzarella, cheddar)
4. Low-fat sour cream
5. Low-fat cream cheese
6. Butter or margarine (low-sodium)
7. Almond or cashew butter (unsweetened)
8. Ricotta cheese (low-fat)
9. Parmesan cheese (grated)

Healthy Fats and Oils:
1. Olive oil
2. Avocado oil
3. Flaxseed oil
4. Coconut oil
5. Nuts (e.g., almonds, walnuts, cashews)
6. Seeds (e.g., chia seeds, flaxseeds, pumpkin seeds)
7. Avocados

Canned and Packaged Goods:
1. Low-sodium canned beans (e.g., black beans, kidney beans, chickpeas)
2. Low-sodium canned tomatoes
3. Low-sodium vegetable broth
4. Low-sodium salsa
5. Whole grain crackers (low-sodium)
6. Rice cakes (unsalted)
7. Whole grain cereal (low-sugar, low-sodium)
8. Unsweetened nut butter (e.g., almond butter, peanut butter)

Herbs, Spices, and Condiments:
1. Garlic
2. Onion
3. Fresh herbs (e.g., basil, parsley, cilantro)
4. Ground spices (e.g., cumin, paprika, turmeric)
5. Salt-free seasoning blends
6. Vinegar (e.g., balsamic vinegar, apple cider vinegar)
7. Low-sodium soy sauce
8. Hot sauce (low-sodium)
9. Mustard (low-sodium)
10. Low-sodium ketchup

11. Salsa (low-sodium)

Beverages:
1. Water
2. Herbal tea (unsweetened)
3. Green tea (unsweetened)
4. Coffee (if permitted)
5. Unsweetened fruit juice (sparingly)

Frozen Foods:
1. Frozen mixed vegetables (low-sodium)
2. Frozen berries (unsweetened)
3. Frozen spinach
4. Frozen broccoli
5. Frozen cauliflower
6. Frozen shrimp or fish fillets (unseasoned, low-sodium)

Snacks:
1. Unsalted nuts (e.g., almonds, pistachios)
2. Unsalted seeds (e.g., sunflower seeds, pumpkin seeds)
3. Rice cakes (unsalted)
4. Low-sodium popcorn
5. Unsweetened applesauce
6. Sugar-free gelatin
7. Low-sodium pretzels
8. Low-sodium crackers

Miscellaneous:
1. Low-sodium cooking spray
2. Unsweetened canned fruit (in water or juice)
3. Low-sodium marinara sauce
4. Low-sodium salsa

5. Low-sodium pasta sauce
6. Low-sodium chicken or vegetable broth

Additional Protein Sources:
1. Lentils
2. Beans (e.g., black beans, kidney beans, chickpeas)
3. Edamame
4. Tempeh
5. Seitan

Additional Vegetables:
1. Asparagus
2. Brussels sprouts
3. Celery
4. Eggplant
5. Mushrooms
6. Onions
7. Peas
8. Squash (e.g., butternut squash, acorn squash)
9. Swiss chard
10. Watercress

CONCLUSION

As we reach the end of "Cooking for Kidney Health: A Diet Cookbook for Men," it's essential to reflect on the journey we've embarked upon together. Through the pages of this cookbook, we've explored the intricacies of kidney disease and its impact on men's health, gaining valuable insights into the importance of dietary adjustments and mindful lifestyle choices in managing this condition.

We've delved into the nuances of crafting a kidney-friendly diet, learning about essential nutrients for optimal kidney health, principles for building balanced and nourishing meals, and practical meal planning tips to simplify healthy eating habits. By embracing these dietary guidelines, men with kidney disease can take proactive steps toward improving their overall well-being and quality of life.

Moreover, we've debunked common myths surrounding exercise for men with kidney disease, highlighting the undeniable physical and mental health benefits of staying active. Through tailored exercise strategies and low-impact workouts, men can enhance their kidney health while fostering strength, resilience, and vitality.

But beyond the recipes and dietary recommendations lies a deeper message of empowerment and resilience. "Cooking for Kidney Health: A Diet Cookbook for Men" is a testament to the strength and determination of men facing the challenges of kidney disease. It's a reminder that with knowledge, support, and a positive mindset, individuals can overcome adversity and thrive despite the obstacles they may encounter.

As you continue your journey toward better kidney health, remember that you're not alone. Whether you're experimenting with new recipes in the kitchen, engaging in gentle exercise routines, or seeking guidance from healthcare professionals, know that there is a community of support rooting for your success every step of the way.

So, as you savor the last bite of your kidney-friendly meal and close the pages of this cookbook, carry with you the lessons learned, the flavors enjoyed, and the hope kindled. May this cookbook serve as a beacon of inspiration and a source of nourishment for your body, mind, and spirit.

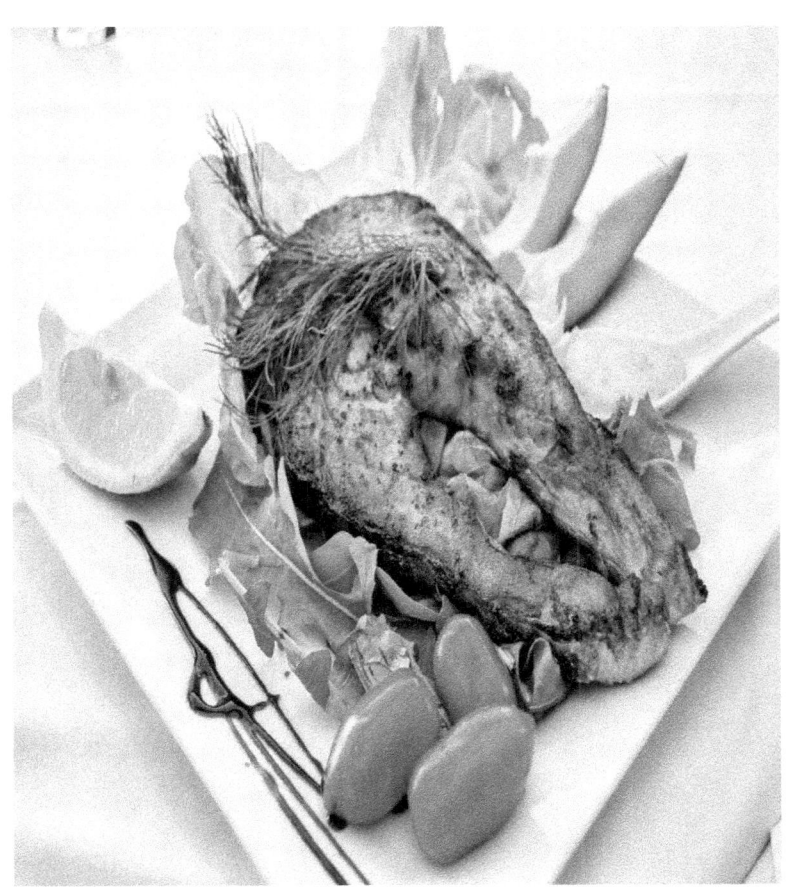

www.ingramcontent.com/pod-product-compliance
Lightning Source LLC
Chambersburg PA
CBHW050318230526
45471CB00005B/2235